LYMPHOMA
PATIENT ADVOCATE

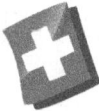

HealthScouter
WWW.HEALTHSCOUTER.COM

HealthScouter.com - Equity Press
5055 Canyon Crest Drive
Riverside, California 92507

www.healthscouter.com

Purchasing this book entitles you to free updates at www.healthscouter.com/Lymphoma

Edited By: Katrina Robinson

Includes Lymphoma from Wikipedia http://en.wikipedia.org/wiki/Lymphoma

Lymphoma

ISBN 978-1-60332-100-6

Important

NEVER DISREGARD PROFESSIONAL MEDICAL ADVICE, OR DELAY SEEKING IT, BECAUSE OF SOMETHING YOU HAVE READ IN THIS BOOK. ALWAYS SEEK PROFESSIONAL MEDICAL ADVICE BEFORE ACTING UPON INFORMATION READ IN THIS BOOK.

HealthScouter and Equity Press do not provide medical advice. The contents of this book are for informational purposes only and are not intended to substitute for professional medical advice, diagnosis or treatment. Always seek advice from a qualified physician or health care professional about any medical concern, and do not disregard professional medical advice because of anything you may read in this book or on a HealthScouter Web site. The views of individuals quoted in this book are not necessarily those of HealthScouter or Equity Press.

While this book is intended to be a medium for the exchange of information and ideas, it is not meant in any way to be a substitute for sound medical advice; neither should it be viewed as a trusted source of such advice. The views expressed in these messages are not those of any qualified medical association, and the publisher is not responsible for the validity of the information communicated herein or for consequences that may arise from acting upon this information. The publisher is not responsible for any content found in the book that may be deemed offensive, inappropriate, inaccurate or medically unsound. The information you find here is only for the purpose of discussion and should not be the basis for any medical decision. The content is not intended to be a substitute for professional medical advice, diagnosis or treatment.

The information presented is not to be considered complete, nor does it contain all medical resource information that may be relevant, and therefore it is not intended to be a substitute for seeking medical treatment and/or appropriate care.

By reading this book and parts of the Web site, you agree under all circumstances to hold harmless, and to refrain from seeking remedy from, the owners of this book. The publisher shall disclaim all liability to you for damages, costs or expenses, including legal and medical fees, related to your reliance on anything derived from this book or Web site or its contents. Furthermore, Equity Press assumes no liability for any and all claims arising out of the said use, regardless of the cause, effects, or fault.

Equity Press and HealthScouter do not endorse any company or product, and listing on the HealthScouter Web site is not linked to corporate sponsorship. We do not make a claim to being comprehensive or up to date. If you would like to recommend information to include in this book, please contact us – we would be very happy to hear from you.

Purchasing this book entitles you to free updates as they are available. Please register your book at www.healthscouter.com

TABLE OF CONTENTS

INTRODUCTION AND MOTIVATION

Dear Reader,

I like to think of myself as a polite, well-reasoned person. I rarely speak out or complain. When a waitress spills something on me, or if my meal is cold—or if I'm overcharged—I generally try to be as polite as possible. I don't like to make very many waves. I often secretly hope that the manager will hear about my predicament and come out and offer me a free meal, or something similar. I generally hope that my polite and respectful demeanor pays off. And it does happen from time to time. You know, I think many people are brought up to believe that this is just good manners. It's how you're supposed to behave. And if you knew me personally, I think you'd agree that I'm generally pretty reserved. Of course my wife may raise an objection or two (!), but I really believe that it's important to treat others as you would like to be treated. We're talking about the golden rule here—it works well and it applies to almost every life circumstance.

But I have to admit that when it comes to my health, or the health of someone I care about—all bets are off. I want to know what's going on—when, why, where, and how. And I make these feelings known. I tend to get downright assertive. It's just something I feel very strongly about. And I feel that when you are in a hospital, or if you're brushing up against the healthcare system, that you should feel the same way. It's unfamiliar turf, and the professionals who work in this system often take advantage of their positions. They may use some jargon to hide the whole truth— or they may say something without checking to make sure you understand completely. They may present the options that are best for them, perhaps the most profitable or convenient. Now I'm not saying this goes on everywhere. There are many professionals in the business of health who go out of their way to make sure you have the best care. And I'm not suggesting that you should become a bully, or purposefully annoying—absolutely not. But I am suggesting that I think it's OK for you to step outside of your typical comfort zone, and put on your patient advocate hat. Because you, the patient or patient advocate, care the most about your care—not the medical system or healthcare providers.

HealthScouter was created to help patients become better advocates for their own medical care. Because when it comes to your healthcare, the stakes are high. There are none higher. And healthcare is one area where consumers (us, the sick people) are notoriously unaware of their options. And that's why I'm publishing these books. To help you understand your options, and to help you get the best care possible. I want to help you become a better advocate for yourself and for your loved ones.

It's my sincere hope that you can take this book with you to the hospital, to be read in the waiting room or by the bedside—and when you see a relevant patient comment you can use this book to ask questions of your health care providers. My advice: Ask lots of questions! Providers are busy people who generally go about their business with little questioning, delivering care as they see fit—making quick decisions—and again, nobody is going to care as much about your health as you. So now, more than ever, you need tools at your disposal to get the best care possible. One of the tools at your disposal is this HealthScouter book and the material within. You need to be armed with questions, and you need to ask questions all of the time. And so the difficult part is now to understand the right questions to ask.

That brings me to an explanation of how these books are structured. HealthScouter books include a number of what we call patient comments. These patient comments are summaries of what people have experienced. They're first hand accounts of what you may expect. These experiences effectively help you "catch up," and understand what outcomes are possible. They expose you to the treatments are available, and provide insight as to potential outcomes. They help you understand what other people are doing. So if you find yourself stuck feeling like you're receiving substandard medical care—or if you need a push to broach the subject, you can take this book to your provider and say, "Hey, I read here that another patient had this treatment—is that an option for me? If not, Why?" I believe that other peoples' experience is the most valuable way for you to formulate and build a list of good questions for your healthcare providers.

That notion is at the core of the HealthScouter philosophy.

So HealthScouter, by providing patient comments about a particular medical condition, will help expose you to what other people have experienced about a particular medical problem. If you know what other people have experienced, you can better understand what your options are. You'll be better informed and you'll have some questions to ask—it'll be like you've had access to dozens of other people who have gone through the same thing you're going through. And so armed, maybe you'll be able to move through your condition and get back on the road to health, and maybe you'll be able to do this with more grace than I have. And that is my sincere wish.

It's also my wish that perhaps when a doctor or nurse sees this little blue book, that they'll think twice about the care they're about to provide—knowing that the owner is a little bit better prepared, a little bit better armed—and yes, maybe even downright assertive.

I hope this book helps.

Yours truly,

Jim Stewart

San Diego, California

HOW TO USE THIS BOOK

The purpose of HealthScouter is to help you understand your medical condition as quickly and easily as possible. We believe this can best be accomplished by reading about other people and their experiences negotiating their health and care. We try to leave out complicated medical jargon. And we've spent a considerable amount of time structuring this book so that it's easy to use. It's important to know that this is not the sort of book you read from beginning to end. Of course you may do so, but this book is more meaningful if you flip through quickly and scan for applicable material. Again, it's all about the patient commentary: The darkly shaded comments ▓ indicate one patient initiating a new discussion, and the light or clear comments ▢ are other comments associated with that same condition. So you should begin by looking for information from other patients who are experiencing the same aspect of the same medical condition that you studying. You can do this quickly by scanning through the book, focusing on the dark shaded comment boxes. By scanning the patient comments you'll find information about various aspects of a condition, all grouped together, in an easy-to-read format. In this way you can immediately begin reading about other patients and their experiences with your particular medical condition – and you can benefit immediately from their experiences.

INTRODUCTION TO LYMPHOMA

Lymphoma is a type of cancer that originates in lymphocytes of the immune system. They often originate in lymph nodes, presenting as an enlargement of the node (a tumour). Lymphomas are closely related to lymphoid leukemias, which also originate in lymphocytes but typically involve only circulating blood and the bone marrow (where blood cells are generated in a process termed haematopoesis) and do not usually form static tumours.[1] There are many types of lymphomas, and in turn, lymphomas are a part of the broad group of diseases called hematological neoplasms.

Thomas Hodgkin published in 1832 the first description of lymphoma, specifically of the form named after him, Hodgkin's lymphoma.[2] Since then many other forms of lymphoma have been described, grouped under several proposed classifications. The 1982 Working formulation classification became very popular. It introduced the category non-Hodgkin lymphoma (NHL), itself divided into 16 different diseases. However, since these different lymphomas have little in common with each other, the non-Hodgkin lymphoma label is of limited usefulness for doctors or patients and is slowly being abandoned. The latest classification by the WHO (2001) lists 43 different forms of lymphoma divided in four broad groups.

Some forms of lymphoma are indolent (e.g. small lymphocytic lymphoma), compatible with a long life even without treatment, whereas other forms are aggressive (e.g. Burkitt's lymphoma), causing rapid deterioration and death. The prognosis therefore depends on the correct classification of the disease, established by a pathologist after examination of a biopsy.[3]

Although older classifications referred to histiocytic lymphomas, these are recognized in newer classifications as of B, T or natural killer cell lineage. True histiocytic malignancies are rare and are classified as sarcomas.[4]

The doctor sent me for some blood test and after a nightmare wait they all came back normal. I was so relieved. That was about a month ago, and as the lumps are still both swollen, I thought it best to go back to the doctor. She told me to leave it for another month, as the blood tests were fine. She said that if the lumps are still there then, she will send me in for an X-ray.

I have to go against what the doctor is telling you and insist that just because blood work results come back normal does not mean a person does not have lymphoma. In the majority of cases when the lump appears, it can be at the beginning stage. The only time the blood tests will show something is when the lymphoma has affected the bone marrow and even then they will probably suspect causes other than lymphoma.

I am a 22 year old female, just looking for some advice and/or reassurance. I found a painless swollen lymph node under my left armpit two weeks ago. It is about 1.5 cm in size and is moveable. It is also not visible from the outside. I spoke to a doctor when I found this! The doctor told me not too worry, to leave it alone and check it in two weeks time and if it's still there go in and see her. I wasn't very good at leaving it alone as I have been so worried about it. Yesterday I went to the doctor's. The doctor gave me a breast examination and said it feels ok and she is not particularly worried about it. She told me again to check in two weeks as it should go down. If still there in two weeks, she will look into it further. I cannot stop worrying about it, and I spend hours searching for different possibilities on the internet. I have no other symptoms, except occasionally I have a twitching feeling (which I can only describe as a baby moving) in my lower stomach. It is not at all painful, and it mainly happens at night. Could this maybe be my spleen swelling?

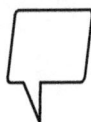

We always tend to think the worst, especially when we find a lump on our body. We hear so much about cancer so that's the first thing we think of. The best thing you did for yourself and your family was going to the doctorr immediately. Those lumps under the armpit can be normal especially because it is an area where us women shave, though they can also be abnormal. I think, if you still have the lump you should go for a second opinion.

I have had two large lymph nodes on either side of my neck towards the base. I have felt them for over 10 years. (I am 24 now.) They are soft and moveable and do not hurt. Lately, however, I have become aware of some lymph nodes in the collar bone area on the right side of my body. I am rather thin, so I am hoping that these are normal. I will make a doctor's appointment on Monday, but what do others think? I do not have any "b" symptoms-night sweats, loss of appetite, etc., but I am still concerned. Also, should I make an appointment with an internist, or my regular *doctor? Should I go straight to someone who knows more about lymphoma or cancer?*

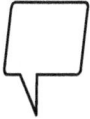

Go to your regular doctor. They will direct you to a specialist if need be.

PREVALENCE

According to the U.S. National Institutes of Health, lymphomas account for about five percent of all cases of cancer in the United States, and Hodgkin's lymphoma in particular accounts for less than one percent of all cases of cancer in the United States.

Because the whole system is part of the body's immune system, patients with a weakened immune system, such as from Human Immunodeficiency Virus infection or from certain drugs or medication, also have a higher incidence of lymphoma.

I have a swollen lymph node on the left side of my neck behind my ear on that long muscle. It's the only one I have. I am not sick aside from seasonal allergies that bring stuffiness, drainage and puffy eyes. Could this be the cause? I'm really worried. It's been this way since Christmas. It did go down in size when I was taking steroids and antibiotics but soon came back.

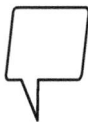

I have a similar problem. I have a swollen lymph node on my neck over my carotid artery. I had an ultrasound done and the lymph node looked normal, but the only way to be sure is a biopsy. I had three fine needle biopsies on it and none of

them reached the node and only drew blood. I have to pay a huge co-pay for a failed procedure. Now my only alternative is an ultrasound-guided biopsy. I have no symptoms of any kind other than the swollen lymph node. I have read that lymph nodes can become swollen due to a virus and never return to their normal size.

CLASSIFICATION

Kiel classification

As an alternative to the American Lukes-Butler classification, in the early 1970s, Karl Lennert proposed a new system of classifying lymphomas based on cellular morphology and their relationship to cells of the normal peripheral lymphoid system.

REAL classification

In the mid 1990s, the Revised European-American Lymphoma (REAL) Classification attempted to apply immunophenotypic and genetic features in identifying distinct clinicopathologic non-Hodgkin lymphoma entities.[5]

WHO classification

The WHO Classification, published in 2001 and updated in 2008,[4] is the latest classification of lymphoma and is based upon the foundations laid within the "Revised European-American Lymphoma classification" (REAL). This system attempts to group lymphomas by cell type (i.e. the normal cell type that most resembles the tumour) and defining phenotypic, molecular or cytogenetic characteristics. There are three large groups: the B cell, T cell, and natural killer cell tumours. Other less common groups are also recognized. Hodgkin's lymphoma, although considered separately within the WHO (and preceding) classifications, is now recognised as being a tumour of, albeit markedly abnormal, lymphocytes of mature B cell lineage.

MATURE B CELL NEOPLASMS

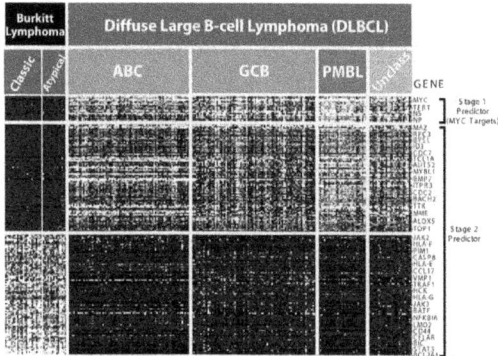

DNA-microarray analysis of Burkitt's lymphoma and diffuse large B-cell lymphoma (DLBCL) showing differences in gene expression patterns. Colors indicate levels of expression; light tones indicate genes that are underexpressed in lymphoma cells (as compared to normal cells), whereas dark tones indicate genes that are overexpressed in lymphoma cells.

- Chronic lymphocytic leukemia/Small lymphocytic lymphoma

- B-cell prolymphocytic leukemia

- Lymphoplasmacytic lymphoma (such as Waldenström macroglobulinemia)

- Splenic marginal zone lymphoma

- Plasma cell neoplasms:

  - Plasma cell myeloma

  - Plasmacytoma

- Monoclonal immunoglobulin deposition diseases

- Heavy chain diseases

- Extranodal marginal zone B cell lymphoma, also called MALT lymphoma

- Nodal marginal zone B cell lymphoma (NMZL)

- Follicular lymphoma

- Mantle cell lymphoma

- Diffuse large B cell lymphoma

- Mediastinal (thymic) large B cell lymphoma

- Intravascular large B cell lymphoma

- Primary effusion lymphoma

- Burkitt lymphoma/leukemia

My dad has just begun CHOP-R chemotherapy for follicular lymphoma (B cell). He was diagnosed a year ago, and other chemotherapy treatments haven't been effective. He retains fluid in his belly and eventually the swelling affects his feet. He has no other significant symptoms of the lymphoma, except that he retains so much fluid and then has to have his abdomen drained with a needle. He was given the CHOP through a line in the hospital for 48 continuous hours. Has anyone had CHOP-R (with rituxan) treatments with good results? And what kind of side effects can we expect?

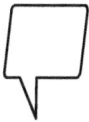

The prednisone can cause edema. Cut way back on salt. The prednisone can lead to diabetes-like conditions. Cut back on high GI foods. The Adriamycin (hydroxydoxorubicin), a.k.a. red devil, can damage the heart. Take melatonin and CoQ10.

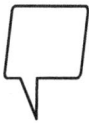

R-CHOP is very harsh. It is also accumulative, meaning symptoms worsen over the course of treatment.

Mature T cell and natural killer (NK) cell neoplasms

- T cell prolymphocytic leukemia

- T cell large granular lymphocytic leukemia

- Aggressive natural killer cell leukemia

- Adult T cell leukemia/lymphoma

- Extranodal natural killer/T cell lymphoma, nasal type

- Enteropathy-type T cell lymphoma

- Hepatosplenic T cell lymphoma

- Blastic natural killer cell lymphoma

- Mycosis fungoides / Sezary syndrome

- Primary cutaneous CD30-positive T cell lymphoproliferative disorders

  - Primary cutaneous anaplastic large cell lymphoma

  - Lymphomatoid papulosis

- Angioimmunoblastic T cell lymphoma

- Peripheral T cell lymphoma, unspecified

- Anaplastic large cell lymphoma

My best friend (age 34 with two small children) was diagnosed with a very rare and aggressive T-cell lymphoma. She has tumors that have turned into big open sores on her legs. The tumor sores weep fluid and smell terrible. She thought the smell was from dead rotting tissue, so she dug it out with a pair of scissors. She now has three deep holes in her leg. She is suddenly VERY weak and tired all the time.

It has been nine months since she was first diagnosed and she has never gone back to the

doctor for a follow up visit or any treatment.
What is really sad is that at her very first doctor
appointment, the oncologist told her that he
wanted to watch it and see what was going to
happen because at the time - all of her CT/MRI
scans were clean and the doctor told her that
she was lacking the "markers" that made it
malignant. She just had these little tiny lumps
in her legs. He wanted to see her four months
later to make sure, because they can change
and become malignant. By then the tumors had
become big sores and when her appointment
came, she cancelled it. She did this because she is
a believer in natural methods and does not want
to do chemotherapy. She is doing this on her own
and I am very scared about that. She is telling
her family that she doesn't have cancer and that
it was all benign. Do I go behind her back and
contact her family and tell them the truth? Would
that be betraying my friend - or should her family
know?

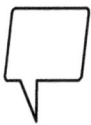

I would most definitely tell her family if you think
they could persuade her to go back to see her
doctor. No-one likes to betray a friend, but I think
because this situation is so serious and probably
life-threatening, you have no choice. Your friend

will most likely be very angry with you, but if you explain that you would prefer to lose her friendship than her lose her life, she might eventually forgive you.

My husband has just been diagnosed with mycosis fungoides stage IA. It's a cutaneous t-cell lymphoma. I just thought I'd try and see if anyone here has this, and how their treatment is going. From what I read, there's no cure, and if caught early, most people live a normal life span, fighting it along the way with creams and other treatments, like puva.

Mycosis fungoides is not a skin cancer, but a type of indolent lymphoma that shows up on the skin rather than attacking the internal organs like other lymphomas. It is a rare disease and very treatable. Because it is rare, it is suggested that patients seek out a specialist for a consultation.

Hodgkin lymphoma

- Classical Hodgkin lymphomas:
  - Nodular sclerosis
  - Mixed cellularity
  - Lymphocyte-rich

- Lymphocyte depleted or not depleted

- Nodular lymphocyte-predominant Hodgkin lymphoma

My husband noticed a lump under his arm about one year ago. After going to the doctor, they said he could leave it there if it didn't bother him. So he left it there. Well last month he woke up with chest pain; in the emergency room, they said he had a minor heart attack. During the week off from work, he decided to get the lump removed. A week after that, we were informed he had Hodgkin's lymphoma, the Nodular Predominant type. After seeing the oncologist and beginning his treatment, we were informed it has spread to his neck, chest and pelvis. We are waiting for the results of the spinal MRI. Any idea how to go through this type of Hodgkin's?

I assume it is Nodular Lymphocyte Predominant Hodgkin's Disease? This is the form that I have, and it is one of the rarest (approx 5%). I do not know what you have read already, but nodular lymphocyte predominant Hodgkin's disease is really a form of non-Hodgkin's lymphoma. Like Classical Hodgkin's disease, nodular lymphocyte predominant Hodgkin's disease affects mainly younger adults, but does not show the second peak in people over the age of 60. If it is just an isolated lymph node, or very few lymph nodes, and there are no other symptoms (Stage 1A), it is treated with radiation therapy alone in the first instance. Sometimes Stage 2 A is also treated like this, although they may recommend a reduced course of chemotherapy as well. If it is more advanced, it is treated with chemotherapy. From the description you give, your husband is Stage 3 if no other organs are involved. The A/B refers to whether he is showing systemic symptoms, such as night sweats, weight loss, itching, pain on consuming alcohol. These symptoms are less common with nodular lymphocyte predominant Hodgkin's disease than with Classical Hodgkin's disease. It is a very slow-growing lymphoma, possibly the slowest.

It will probably be treated with a combination of drugs known as ABVD. However, the link with non-Hodgkin's comes in here, and some centers are now adding Rituximab, which is a mono-clonal antibody therapy, so it becomes R-ABVD. Rituximab has been used to very good effect with non-Hodgkin's lymphoma, where the chemo used is R-CHOP. It has not been studied extensively

*in nodular lymphocyte predominant Hodgkin's
disease, so it is not known to what extent it gives
an advantage over standard chemotherapy. The
good thing about it is that, so far as we know,
there are rarely any side-effects, so the patient is
unlikely to feel any worse than they would with
standard chemo.*

*The majority of people with nodular lymphocyte
predominant Hodgkin's disease are cured by
treatment, i.e. they have their treatment and are
not bothered by the disease again.*

Immunodeficiency-associated lymphoproliferative disorders

- Associated with a primary immune disorder

- Associated with the Human Immunodeficiency
  Virus (HIV)

- Post-transplant

- Associated with Methotrexate therapy

Working formulation and Non-Hodgkin lymphoma

The 1982 Working Formulation is a classification
of Non-Hodgkin Lymphoma. It has since been
replaced by other lymphoma classifications, the
latest published by the WHO in 2001 (updated in

September 2008), but is still used by cancer agencies for compilation of lymphoma statistics.

Other classification systems

- ICD-O (codes 9590-9999, details at [1]) (archive link, was dead)

- ICD-10 (codes C81-C96, details at [2])

LYMPHOID LEUKEMIA

Lymphoid leukemia (*Lymphoid* meaning lymphoma like) (or lymphocytic leukemia) is a type of leukemia affecting circulating cells of lymphoid origin. This is in contrast to lymphoma, which is a solid tumor of lymphoid cells.[1]

Classification

Historically, they have been most commonly divided by the stage of maturation at which the clonal (neoplastic) lymphoid population stopped maturing:

• Acute lymphoblastic leukemia

• Chronic lymphocytic leukemia

However, the influential WHO Classification (published in 2001) emphasized a greater emphasis on cell lineage. To this end, lymphoid leukemias can also be divided by the type of cells affected:

• T-cell leukemia

• B-cell leukemia

HODGKIN'S LYMPHOMA

Hodgkin's lymphoma, also known as Hodgkin's disease, is a type of lymphoma (cancer originating from a type of white blood cells called lymphocytes). It was named after Thomas Hodgkin, who first described abnormalities in the lymph system in 1832.[1]

Hodgkin's lymphoma is characterized by the orderly spread of disease from one lymph node group to another, and by the development of systemic symptoms with advanced disease. The disease is characterized by the presence of Reed-Sternberg cells (RS cells) on microscopic examination. Hodgkin lymphoma was one of the first cancers which could be treated using radiation therapy and, later, it was one of the first to be treated by combination chemotherapy.

The disease occurrence shows two peaks: the first in young adulthood (age 15–35) and the second in those over 55 years old. The survival rate is generally 90% or higher when the disease is detected during early stages, making it one of the more curable forms of cancer.[2] Hodgkin's lymphoma is one of the handful of cancers that, even in its later stages, has a very high cure rate, in the 90's.[3]

Most patients who are able to be successfully treated (and thus enter remission) generally go on and live long and normal lives, due to a remission success rate of 90% to 95%.

I keep reading that one of the symptoms of lymphoma is itchy skin. For the past few months, my legs would itch. I thought it was dry skin, so I would put lotion on it and benadryl. It would take a long time for anything to stop the itching. I was brushing my teeth a few weeks ago and my left hand starting to itch. I had never felt anything like it before. Then a blue lump (bruise) appeared and hurt very badly. I thought it was a blood vessel or clot. After about 1/2 hour, it stopped, and eventually the bruise went away. My brother had Hodgkin's. Is it hereditary?

With your family history, you have every reason to feel nervous. It sounds like you are having all kinds of symptoms because you are so stressed out from worrying. That kind of stress can do you more harm than anything! Find a doctor ASAP and ask them their opinion.

Lymphoma has many symptoms and it doesn't mean that everyone with lymphoma has the same symptoms or any of them for that matter. When a person has lymphoma without symptoms, they are classified as the type of lymphoma. Those who do have lymphoma and symptoms are classified with the type of lymphoma plus the letter B next to it. This indicates that they have symptoms. The itchy skin and night sweats are common symptoms, and the fact that you have an enlarged lymph node on your armpit should raise a red flag. I would insist on a biopsy of that node; you will get guaranteed answers.

To answer your question "is Hodgkin's hereditary?": not always, though it is more common amongst siblings.

I have felt my ENTIRE body. No lumps, no swollen lymph nodes. The only symptom I have is a weird body rash that comes out of nowhere usually at night and goes away after like ten minutes. I keep hearing that's a symptom of lymphoma. Am I just being paranoid?

You can really make yourself sick just from worrying. You can get a rash from your nerves, an itchy red rash. Dry skin can cause your skin to itch all over. I can't say enough to you to not stress out.

Classification

Types

Classical Hodgkin's lymphoma (excluding nodular lymphocyte predominant Hodgkin's lymphoma) can be subclassified into four pathologic subtypes based upon Reed-Sternberg cell morphology and the composition of the reactive cell infiltrate seen in the lymph node biopsy specimen (the cell composition around the Reed-Stenberg cell(s)).

Do you happen to know how many types of Hodgkin's there are?

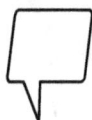

Hodgkin's tends to be divided into classical Hodgkin's and Lymphocyte Predominant, which only accounts for about 5% of cases. The latter is now considered not to be a true form of Hodgkin's at all, because it does not have the characteristic Reed-Sternberg giant cells, which are diagnostic of Hodgkin's. It does have large cells, called popcorn cells, which can look similar to Reed-Sternberg cells, probably explaining why it was originally classified as a form of Hodgkin's. The progression of the disease tends to be very indolent (slow), whereas classical Hodgkin's tends to be quite aggressive, so many people believe it should be

reclassified as a form of low grade non-Hodgkin's lymphoma. However, like classical Hodgkin's, the age of onset of lymphocyte predominant tends to be in the twenties and thirties, it often presents with an enlarged lymph node in the neck, and it responds to the same types of chemotherapy as forms of classical Hodgkin's. Usually, if caught early, the prognosis is similar to classical Hodgkin's. However, if you are unfortunate enough to relapse, it acts more like a low-grade non-Hodgkin's, i.e. it responds to treatment again, but tends to come back and keep coming back. Unlike classical Hodgkin's, where relapses are most common in the first two years, and increasingly unlikely as time goes by, the indolent nature of lymphocyte predominant Hodgkin's means it is unlikely to return in the first two years, but more likely to return thereafter.

Classical Hodgkin's is generally divided into four subtypes: lymphocyte rich, nodular sclerosing, lyphocyte depleted and mixed cellularity. Unlike the case with lymphocyte predominant, these are all considered to be different forms of the same disease.

Name	Description	ICD-10	ICD-O
Nodular sclerosing Classical Hodgkin's lymphoma	Is the most common subtype and is composed of large tumor *nodules* showing scattered lacunar classical Reed-Sternberg cells set in a background of reactive lymphocytes, eosinophils and plasma cells with varying degress of collagen fibrosis/*sclerosis*.	C81.1	M9663/3
Mixed-cellularity subtype	Is a common subtype and is composed of numerous classic Reed-Sternberg cells admixed with numerous inflammatory cells including lymphocytes, histiocytes, eosinophils, and plasma cells. without sclerosis. This type is most often associated with EBV infection and may be confused with the early, so-called 'cellular' phase of nodular sclerosing Classical Hodgkin's lymphoma.	C81.2	M9652/3.
Lymphocyte-rich	Is a rare subtype, show many features which may cause diagnostic confusion with nodular lymphocyte predominant B-cell Non-Hodgkin's Lymphoma (B-NHL).	C81.0	M9651/3
Lymphocyte depleted	Is a rare subtype, composed of large numbers of often pleomorphic Reed-Sternberg cells with only few reactive lymphocytes which may easily be confused with diffuse large cell lymphoma. Many cases previously classified within this category would now be reclassified under anaplastic large cell lymphoma.[4]	C81.3	M9653/3
Unspecified		C81.9	M9650/3

Nodular lymphocyte predominant Hodgkin's lymphoma expresses CD20, and is not currently considered a form of classical Hodgkin's.

For the other forms, although the traditional B cell markers (such as CD20) are not expressed on all cells,[4] Reed-Sternberg cells are usually of B cell origin.[5][6] Although Hodgkin's is now frequently grouped with other B cell malignancies, some T cell markers (such as CD2 and CD4) are occasionally expressed.[7] However, this may be an artifact of the ambiguity inherent in the diagnosis.

Hodgkin's cells produce Interleukin-21 (IL-21), which was once thought to be exclusive to T cells. This feature may explain the behavior of classical Hodgkin's lymphoma, including clusters of other immune cells gathered around HL cells (infiltrate) in cultures.[8]

Staging

After Hodgkin's lymphoma is diagnosed, a patient will be *staged:* that is, they will undergo a series of tests and procedures which will determine what areas of the body are affected. These procedures will include documentation of their histology, a physical examination, blood tests, chest X-ray radiographs, computed tomography (CT) scans or magnetic resonance imaging (MRI) scans of the chest, abdomen and pelvis, and a bone marrow biopsy. Positron emission tomography (PET) scan is now used instead of the gallium scan for staging. In the past, a lymphangiogram or surgical laparotomy (which involves opening the abdominal cavity and visually inspecting for tumors) were performed. Lymphangiograms or laparotomies are very rarely performed, having been supplanted by improvements in imaging with the CT scan and PET scan.

On the basis of this staging, the patient will be classified according to a staging classification (the Ann Arbor staging classification scheme is a common one):

- Stage I is involvement of a single lymph node region (I) or single extralymphatic site (Ie);

- Stage II is involvement of two or more lymph node regions on the same side of the diaphragm (II) or of one lymph node region and a contiguous extralymphatic site (IIe);

- Stage III is involvement of lymph node regions on both sides of the diaphragm, which may include the spleen (IIIs) and/or limited contiguous extralymphatic organ or site (IIIe, IIIes);

- Stage IV is disseminated involvement of one or more extralymphatic organs.

The absence of systemic symptoms is signified by adding 'A' to the stage; the presence of systemic symptoms is signified by adding 'B' to the stage. For localized extranodal extension from mass of nodes which does not advance the stage, subscript 'E' is added.

Three weeks ago I had a sharp pain in my right inguinal area. It wasn't until I felt the pain that I felt a lump in my lymph node. I went to my family doctor and they took me right over to have a CT scan. The doctor gave me some pain medicine. He referred me to a specialist for the remaining of this problem. I met with the specialist, and he read me the CT results. 3.4 x 2.5 cm node. He recommended a biopsy. The results stated that the finding were suspicious for lymphoma. Since neither doctor did any type of blood work, I am not sure I want this specialist to cut on me yet. If I do have lymphoma, what should I be looking for? What are the consequences of having a node removed? If it is not Lymphoma, how long for this swelling to go down?

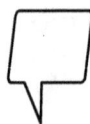

Scans of any type can NOT detect if a mass is a malignancy. ONLY a biopsy can detect a malignancy for sure, and sometimes they are misdiagnosed. So it's always good to always get a second opinion and even a third opinion if the patient wants it.

There are three ways they can biopsy it: they can remove the entire mass, take a piece of the tissue and view it, or do a needle biopsy which is called a fine needle aspiration. I don't see the harm of having the biopsy.

Signs and symptoms

Patients with Hodgkin lymphoma may present with the following symptoms:

• Night Sweats

I don't know what my lymph nodes should feel like. I know I have bumps under my skin, but they are not visible whichever way I turn my neck. They are located right around where you feel your pulse. Also, my right ear has been plugged up, but if I press on my neck on the right side, it goes away. I had three bouts of night sweats but not for a few weeks now. Would these lymph nodes be getting larger? Would the night

sweats have just stopped or would they continue and get worse?

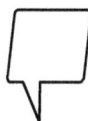

No, the night sweats would not go away. As for the lymph nodes: they can swell if you have a common cold or virus or even with allergies. I really don't think you are showing signs of lymphoma, and I don't even think that your symptoms are related. Go see your general physician for answers.

• Lymph nodes: the most common symptom of Hodgkin's is the painless enlargement of one or more lymph nodes. The nodes may also feel rubbery and swollen when examined. The nodes of the neck and shoulders (cervical and supraclavicular) are most frequently involved (80–90% of the time, on average). The lymph nodes of the chest are often affected and these may be noticed on a chest radiograph.

• Splenomegaly: enlargement of the spleen occurs in about 30% of people with Hodgkin's lymphoma. The enlargement, however, is seldom massive and the size of the spleen may fluctuate during the course of treatment.

- Hepatomegaly: enlargement of the liver, due to liver involvement, is present in about five percent of cases.

- Hepatosplenomegaly: the enlargement of both the liver and spleen caused by the same disease.

- Pain:

- Pain following alcohol consumption: classically, involved nodes are painful after alcohol consumption, though this phenomenon is very uncommon.[9]

- Back pain: nonspecific back pain (pain that cannot be localized or its cause determined by examination or scanning techniques) has been reported in some cases of Hodgkin lymphoma. The lower back is most often affected.

- Red-colored patches on the skin, easy bleeding and petechiae due to low platelet count

- Systemic symptoms: about one-third of patients with Hodgkin's disease may also present with systemic symptoms, including low-grade fever; night sweats; unexplained weight loss of at least 10% of the patient's total body mass in six months or less, itchy skin (pruritus) due to increased levels of eosinophils in the bloodstream; or fatigue (lassitude). Systemic symptoms such as fever, night sweats, and weight loss are known as B symptoms; thus, presence of fever, weight loss, and night sweats indicate that the patient's stage is, for example, 2B instead of 2A.[10]

- Cyclical fever: patients may also present with a cyclical high-grade fever known as the Pel-Ebstein fever,[11] or more simply "P-E fever". However, there is debate as to whether or not the P-E fever truly exists[12].

> *I have had severe itching on my face, neck and both hands for more than three months. My doctor has sent me to a dermatologist, and she gave me hydrocortisone cream and a reactine tablet, but still it is increasing only. For the last two months, I am having pain on my left jaw with swollen lymph nodes. Now pain is spreading to my throat, left side of jaw, and inside my mouth on the gum. Today I explained that to my doctor, but he says lymph node swelling and pain are due to the facial itching and to just take tylenol. But now I am extremely worried after seeing the symptoms of lymphoma in the net. Also now I have realized that I have had night sweating for some time as well as fatigue and weight loss. Please someone tell me*

if this could be lymphoma or it could be allergies and what should I do.

You cannot diagnose anything yourself. What you need to do is go to your doctor and ask for some blood work done. Only after the results can someone really tell you what's going on. Don't read too much online as when you are worried about something, you will fit your symptoms to theirs.

You need to go back to the doctor and insist on the proper tests. If your doctor dismisses you, please seek a second opinion. Blood tests will not tell you if you have lymphoma; you need to get a biopsy of that node. Lymphoma does have the same symptoms as many other diseases; therefore, it's not so simple to diagnose. The fact that you say you have an enlarged node, weight loss, and night sweats is cause for concern. If your doctor sends you for blood work and the results come back normal and he says everything is ok, please insist on a biopsy.

The lymph node in my neck is roughly pea sized and the one under my armpit about baked bean. They have both been that size for about a month and a half. Would they not be getting bigger if it was something more serious?

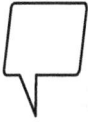

Would they get bigger? Not necessarily. A biopsy is your best bet, it is a simple procedure and will give you answers.

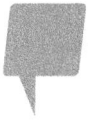

In January, my 40-year-old husband started having night sweats. They got so bad that after a few weeks, we went to the doctors and were sent to see a consultant. He sent him for an ultrasound scan. Half way through the scan, they stopped it and said he needed a CT scan. This was done on his gallbladder. We went back to see the doctor and were told he had sludge in his gallbladder and they would remove it. He was checked for tuberculosis, which was ruled out. When bloods were removed for testing, a massive yellow bruise appeared on his arm which we blamed on the technician's method. He had the operation in March, and the night sweats carried on. He also started having breathing difficulties, which would come on for no apparent reason. They were not unlike the symptoms for asthma. Our general practitioner gave him an inhaler. The next thing was an itching all over his throat. Again we put this down to the asthma or maybe hay fever. Six weeks ago a lump appeared in the middle at the bottom of his back, and the doctor said it was a cyst. He then started to get very tired and lethargic and lost his appetite. Next he started with tummy pains around the site where the gallbladder was removed from his lower back. Last weekend he was very tired and not well at all; the night sweats were bad although he does not get these every night. On Monday a tiny red spot appeared in his chin; it started to bleed and we could not stop it. The other strange thing is his temperature: he is hot one minute and cold the next. On Tuesday we decided it was time to sort this out once and for all.

We made an appointment with the general practitioner. She examined him and said his liver was very enlarged; she also examined his back. When she touched his left side, it was painful. She checked him for swollen glands but did not say if she found any. She said she was very concerned and made us an appointment for Thursday with a specialist.

We arrived for the appointment; the doctor gave him a full examination and took all his history. He then told us that he thought it was Lymphoma. He had blood taken and a full CT scan is booked for Monday. What I am finding hard to believe *is that this could have been missed in March when they removed his gallbladder. How can the doctor come to this diagnosis by just examination and history? How is Lymphoma diagnosed?*

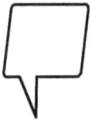

Once they have done the scan to determine where the swollen glands are, he will have a biopsy of the gland. Specific cells they will see on a microscope will tell if it is Hodgkin's or non-Hodgkin's - there is no other way to determine this. They will then (usually) do a bone marrow biopsy to determine whether or not there is involvement there. The staging is usually stage I: nodes affected above the diaphragm; stage II: nodes affected below the diaphragm; stage III: nodes both above and below affected (and any lymphatic organs such as the spleen); and stage IV is when there is also other organ involvement, commonly the liver or the brain and/or bone marrow infiltration. His oncologist/hematologist will then decide what the best treatment is. Some people receive a combination chemotherapy, others both chemo and radiation therapy and some just radiation.

My daughter has a lump under her armpit you can see it by standing about 10 feet away from her. I took her to the doctor, and he found some more enlarged nodes on one side of her neck

and in her groin. They are painless. Has anyone had any of these symptoms?

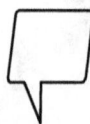

My son was diagnosed with Stage IV Lymphoblastic Lymphoma when he was six years old. There are some things I would like to pass on to you.

1) Always go with your mother's intuition (your gut feeling). It has saved me many times. You know your daughter better than anyone and you know when something is wrong.

2) Don't stop pushing for results. If you don't feel comfortable with your doctor, try and get into another doctor. It never hurts to have a second opinion.

3) Research, research, research.

4) If your daughter does have cancer, there is always hope. My son was given a 70% chance of survival at diagnosis (because his case was so advanced) and when he relapsed (after 18 months of treatment and nine months remission) it went down to 15% without a bone marrow transplant and 20% with a transplant (we opted for the latter). The point is my son is here, he survived.

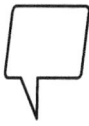

Enlarged lymph nodes can be a sign of a serious illness like Hodgkin's or non Hodgkin's lymphoma. The best thing you and your doctor are doing for your child is that scan. It is important to make the diagnosis as quick as possible in order to treat quickly.

About four months ago I felt a lump on my throat about 1 centimeter, firm, rubbery (not rock hard) and easily moveable. It didn't hurt or feel at all tender. I've of course had swollen lymph nodes before, but never when I wasn't been sick and none that had this sort of consistency. Anyway, I pretty much forgot about it for a few months. Recently, it has gotten a little larger. It is still non-tender and feels like a rubbery marble. A couple of weeks ago, I noticed several lymph nodes in my groin with the same texture. A couple are about a centimeter big and rubbery and a few are very small and hard. All of them move around easily and feel like they are in a chain.

Anyway, this week I went to my doctor for my annual physical and mentioned the lump in my neck. My doctor felt it and said it was a lymph node and that he didn't like the way it felt. He said I should go to an ear, nose and throat doctor to have it looked at. I didn't mention my groin lumps to him because I forgot.

Every since the appointment I have been totally freaked out and panicked.

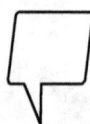

My best suggestion is to call that doctor back, the original one you saw, and tell him you have lymph nodes in the groin area too that can be felt. Maybe you can bypass the upcoming appointment.

Risk factors

There are no guidelines for preventing Hodgkin lymphoma because the cause is unknown. A risk factor is something that statistically increases your chance of getting a disease or condition. Risk factors include:[13]

• Sex: male

• Ages: 15–40 and over 55

• Family history

• History of infectious mononucleosis or infection with Epstein-Barr virus, a causative agent of mononucleosis

- Weakened immune system, including infection with Human Immunodeficiency Virus or the presence of AIDS

- Prolonged use of human growth hormone

Is Hodgkin's disease hereditary?

They believe that if there is a genetic cause, then siblings have a 1% increased chance of developing the disease, but as far as I'm aware, no other relatives have the increased risk. However, they also don't know if it environmental and if it is then chances are most people were brought up in the same area/house as their siblings so if something in the environment has been the cause then it could is likely to be the same for the sibling.

Research has shown that Hodgkin's is not hereditary, though it is very common amongst siblings.

Diagnosis

Hodgkin lymphoma must be distinguished from non-cancerous causes of lymph node swelling (such as various infections) and from other types of cancer. Definitive diagnosis is by lymph node biopsy (Usually excisional biopsy with microscopic examination). Blood tests are also performed to assess function of major organs and to assess safety for chemotherapy. Positron emission tomography (PET) is used to detect small deposits that do not show on CT scanning. In some cases a Gallium Scan may be used instead of a PET scan.

How long does it take to get a biopsy of lymph glands to see if it's cancerous?

My personal experience is that when I had a biopsy done by a pulmonologist as an outpatient, it took 2 1/2 weeks. After they admitted me to the hospital they did another one and it took about seven days. Of course with the second one they basically knew what they were looking for where with the first one they had no idea.

I am having a biopsy on some lymph nodes in my abdomen tomorrow; what can I expect? It is going to hurt?

That depends on the procedure. If it is a needle biopsy, that's minimally invasive, and probably not too painful. If it's a laparoscopy, that's considerably more invasive, and involves them putting air into the abdomen. You'd be a bit sore for a couple of days. If it's a full laparotomy, that's quite a big operation, and you will be sore for a couple of weeks.

I imagine it's a needle biopsy if they are not admitting you for a few days, so minimal discomfort.

I am a 20 year old African American woman, with really no major health concerns besides high blood pressure. But I am very worried about my health now. In August of last year, I had some lower back pain that would come and go for about a month. For the most part, the pain is no longer present.

Then, on September 20, I noticed that the lymph nodes under my arm were swollen. So for around four months, the lymph nodes under my arms have been swollen. Sometimes they hurt a little, and sometimes they don't. I am always touching, poking, and feeling them because they are bothering me and makng me scared.

Then on October 22, I realized that I had a painless lump behind each one of my knees. Mind you, I have had knee problems in the past. The lumps cause no pain at all; you cannot feel them when I am sitting down and can only see or feel them when I stand up or when I am on my tiptoes.

On November 20, I went to the hospital because I wasn't feeling well. My body was jittery and shaky, everyone was telling me that I looked pale, and my lymph nodes under my arm were still swollen after two months. So when I went to the doctor, she felt the lumps behind my knees and my lymph nodes in my underarms, and didn't seem to concern about them.

So then last week, I went to see a blood pressure doctor for a routine check-up. I told her about the lumps in the back of my knees, but just like the other doctors, she didn't concern herself with them.

My questions are, since my lymph nodes under both of my arms are still swollen, should I be worried? Could I possible have lymphoma or some other form of cancer? Can a complete blood count test diagnose lymphoma? Should I make another appointment with my doctor, even though she was not concerned about my swollen lymph nodes before?

A complete blood count test cannot detect lymphoma. You should definitely get those lumps checked; they can be lipomas, which are fatty deposits, but they can be a sign of lymphoma. A biopsy of a node can be the best way to accurately diagnose what's going on; if you're concerned, you should request a PET scan. It is important to get those blood test results because lymphoma also affects your bone marrow.

Pathology

Macroscopy

Affected lymph nodes (most often, laterocervical lymph nodes) are enlarged, but their shape is preserved because the capsule is not invaded. Usually, the cut surface is white-grey and uniform; in some histological subtypes (e.g. nodular sclerosis) a nodular aspect may appear.

Microscopy

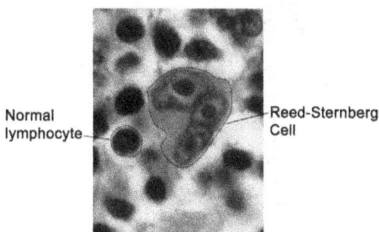

Normal lymphocyte

Reed-Sternberg Cell

Microscopic examination of the lymph node biopsy reveals complete or partial effacement of the lymph node architecture by scattered large malignant cells known as Reed-Sternberg cells (RSC) (typical and variants) admixed within a reactive cell infiltrate composed of variable proportions of lymphocytes, histiocytes, eosinophils, and plasma cells. The Reed-Sternberg cells are identified as large often bi-nucleated cells with prominent nucleoli and an unusual CD45-, CD30+, CD15+/- immunophenotype. In approximately 50% of cases, the Reed-Sternberg cells are infected by the Epstein-Barr virus. Characteristics of classic Reed-Sternberg cells include large size (20–50 micrometres), abundant, amphophilic, finely granular/homogeneous cytoplasm; two mirror-image nuclei (owl eyes) each with an eosinophilic nucleolus and a thick nuclear membrane (chromatin is distributed at the cell periphery).

Variants:

- Hodgkin cell (atypical mononuclear Reed-Sternberg Cell) is a variant of Reed-Sternberg cell, which has the same characteristics, but is mononucleated.

- Lacunar Reed-Sternberg Cell is large, with a single hyperlobated nucleus, multiple, small nucleoli and eosinophilic cytoplasm which is retracted around the nucleus, creating an empty space ("lacunae").

- Pleomorphic Reed-Sternberg Cell has multiple irregular nuclei.

- "Popcorn" Reed-Sternberg Cell (lympho-histiocytic variant) is a small cell, with a very lobulated nucleus, small nucleoli.

- "Mummy" Reed-Sternberg Cell has a compact nucleus, no nucleolus and basophilic cytoplasm.

Hodgkin's lymphoma can be sub-classified by histological type. The cell histology in Hodgkin's lymphoma is not as important as it is in non-Hodgkin's lymphoma: the treatment and prognosis in classic Hodgkin's lymphoma usually depends on the stage of disease rather than the histotype.

I'm a year and three months in remission from Hodgkin's Lymphoma 2A. I have a CT scan every three months, and soon will start every four months-- then it continues until five years---which I'm told then, they'll say I'm "cured." I have to have a gallstone removed. Do you think there's a possibility that I could have my gallstone and my port removed at the same time? I asked my chemo nurse that question, the last time I had my port flushed, and she said she would look into it. When is the "normal" time to have a port removed?

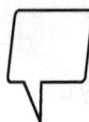

I am surprised that you still have your port in. Everyone I know, and this is in the United Kingdom bear in mind rather than the United States, has their port taken out pretty soon after they finish treatment. I understand that they are keeping it in just in case, but I would have thought the risk of infection outweighed the benefits of not having to fit another in the event of a relapse. If it gets infected, they will have to take it out anyway: this happened to a friend of mine.

I am a physically fit 17-year-old male who plays sports. I am very skinny. I don't drink or smoke and I get plenty of sleep and eat well. For about five years, I've been able to feel many lymph nodes in my neck and groin area. About eight weeks ago, I noticed some slight yellow coloration in the whites of my eyes under the eyelids. I noticed that my leg hairs had become frizzier. I don't think I'm losing any hair, but I'm able to pluck hair with no pain. I had some blood work done a week ago and I found out my bilirubin level is 3.0H mg/dL (the normal range is 0.1–1.2). The doctor thinks it is probably Gilbert's

Syndrome. I had an ultrasound soon after and discovered that I have lymph nodes around the body of my pancreas and aorta. At least one of these lymph nodes is 2.06 cm. The doctors don't seem too worried, and I am scheduled to have a needle biopsy of my lymph nodes tomorrow.

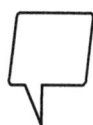

The best thing that you can be doing right now is having that biopsy. It is a simple procedure that will give you the answers you're looking for. Enlarged nodes and the fact that the bilirubin level is above the normal range can be a number of things. Make sure your doctor rules out Hodgkin's lymphoma or non-Hodgkin's lymphoma. People with lymphoma do have similar symptoms as you.

Prognosis

Treatment of Hodgkin's disease has been improving over the past few decades. Recent trials that have made use of new types of chemotherapy have indicated higher survival rates than have previously been seen. In one recent European trial, the 5-year survival rate for those patients with a favorable prognosis was 98%, while that for patients with worse outlooks was at least 85%.[2]

In 1998, an international effort[14] identified seven prognostic factors that accurately predict the success rate of conventional treatment in patients with locally extensive or advanced stage Hodgkin's lymphoma. Freedom from progression (FFP) at 5 years was directly related to the number of factors present in a patient. The 5-year freedom from progression for patients with zero factors is 84%. Each additional factor lowers the 5-year freedom from progression rate by 7%, such that the 5-year freedom from progression for a patient with 5 or more factors is 42%.

The adverse prognostic factors identified in the international study are:

- Age $\geq$ 45 years

- Stage IV disease

- Hemoglobin <10.5 g/dl

- Lymphocyte count <600/µl or <8%

- Male

- Albumin <4.0 g/dl

- White blood count $\geq$ 15,000/µl

Other studies have reported the following to be the most important adverse prognostic factors: mixed-cellularity or lymphocyte-depleted histologies, male sex, large number of involved nodal sites, advanced stage, age of 40 years or more, the presence of B symptoms, high erythrocyte sedimentation rate, and bulky disease (widening of the mediastinum by more than one third, or the presence of a nodal mass measuring more than 10 cm in any dimension.)

Is lymphoma curable? I thought it was like leukemia where just about everyone dies.

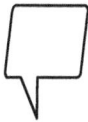

Many patients with lymphoma have treatment and are cured, i.e. the lymphoma goes away and does not come back. So yes, it is curable. Unfortunately, this is not everyone.

I think the same is true of leukemia. Many patients have their treatment; the problem goes away and does not come back. So this is also curable, but the treatments still do not cure everybody.

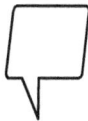

It really depends on which lymphoma you have. Some are curable; some are treatable but not curable. Those are the indolent ones that develop slowly. However, with more treatments coming on board and longer remissions. there is hope that all types will eventually become curable.

Treatment

Patients with early stage disease (IA or IIA) are effectively treated with radiation therapy or chemotherapy. The choice of treatment depends on the age, sex, bulk and the histological subtype of the disease. Patients with later disease (III, IVA, or IVB) are treated with combination chemotherapy alone. Patients of any stage with a large mass in the chest are usually treated with combined chemotherapy and radiation therapy.

I wonder if there are other survivors who are experiencing some of the long term effects of the chemotherapy. I had MOPP/ABVD regime. I was in stage 4 with tumors in lining of heart and lungs. I have started having various health problems and I suspect are due to the chemotherapy. I have just developed tachycardia with left atrial enlargement, my pituitary gland is not functioning properly, constant ringing in my ears, and have had to have extensive dental work due to the radiation. I am curious if there are other long term survivors who have experienced long term effects of chemotherapy and radiation.

I, too, had Hodgkin's and am in remission. I had ABVD (eight treatments) and 20 rad's. I had no idea about the repercussions that would follow. This first year after treatment, I experienced aches, breathing problems, stomach ulcers, acid reflux, gallstones, and anemia. When you compare it to the alternative, I suppose it's not that bad.

From my earlier chemo, which was ClVPP, a MOPP variant, I made a good recovery, but have had some ongoing problems. My digestive system never recovered fully, and I have endured IBS-type symptoms ever since. I have also had ongoing problems with fissures at the output end of the system - they can really hurt. For years now, my doctors have predicted thyroid problems, which have thankfully not emerged. Blood tests show thyroid function to be borderline at times, but so far it has always bounced back again. I do get episodes of tachycardia, but that is a recent thing, which I attribute to the R-ABVD. That seems to be settling down now though. This regime has hit me hard, but it's my second lot of chemotherapy, and I'm 11 years older than the first time. Too early to say what the long-term effects will be.

ABVD	Stanford V	BEACOPP
Currently, the ABVD chemotherapy regimen is the gold standard for treatment of Hodgkin's disease. The abbreviation stands for the four drugs Adriamycin, bleomycin, vinblastine, and dacarbazine. Developed in Italy in the 1970s, the ABVD treatment typically takes between six and eight months, although longer treatments may be required.	Another form of treatment is the newer Stanford V regimen, which is typically only half as long as the ABVD but which involves a more intensive chemotherapy schedule and incorporates radiation therapy. However, in a randomized controlled study, Stanford V was inferior. [15]	Another form of treatment, mainly in Europe for stages >II is BEACOPP. The cure rate with the BEACOPP esc. regimen is approximately 10–15% higher than with standard ABVD in advanced stages. Although this was shown in a landmark paper in The New England Journal of Medicine (Diehl *et al.*), the US physicians still favor ABVD, which may be because some physicians think that BEACOPP induces more secondary leukemia. However, this seems negligible compared to the higher cure rates. Also, BEACOPP is more expensive because of the requirement for concurrent treatment with GCSF to increase production of white blood cells. Currently, the German Hodgkin Study Group tests 8 cycles (8x) BEACOPP esc vs. 6x BEACOPP esc vs. 8x BEACOPP-14 baseline (HD15-trial). [16]
Doxorubicin	Doxorubicin	Doxorubicin
Bleomycin	Bleomycin	Bleomycin
Vinblastine	Vinblastine, Vincristine	Vincristine
Dacarbazine	Mechlorethamine	Cyclophosphamide, Procarbazine
	Etoposide	Etoposide
	Prednisone	Prednisone

Although increased age is an adverse risk factor for Hodgkin's lymphoma, in general elderly patients without major comorbidities are sufficiently fit to tolerate standard therapy, and have a treatment outcome comparable to that of younger patients. However, the disease is a different entity in older patients and different considerations enter into treatment decisions.[17]

The high cure rates and long survival of many patients with Hodgkin's lymphoma has led to a high concern with late adverse effects of treatment, including cardiovascular disease and second malignancies such as acute leukemias, lymphomas, and solid tumors within the radiation therapy field. Most patients with early stage disease are now treated with abbreviated chemotherapy and involved-field radiation therapy rather than with radiation therapy alone. Clinical research strategies are exploring reduction of the duration of chemotherapy and dose and volume of radiation therapy in an attempt to reduce late morbidity and mortality of treatment while maintaining high cure rates. Hospitals are also treating those who respond quickly to chemotherapy with no radiation.

My husband had stage 2A Hodgkin's about 15 years ago. He went through a year of chemotherapy. Can he have kids? Are there any success stories here?

Many men that have done chemotherapy cannot conceive a child, though it does not mean all. Usually, when a man still wants to have children before having chemotherapy he is asked if he wants to freeze his sperm because it is not for sure if he will be able to conceive after treatments. He can consult his physicians and they will be able to check him and find out. If he doesn't want to, then the best way is to try to conceive that'll be the sure way of finding out.

I am a mom of an adult daughter who was diagnosed last week with Hodgkin's. She will be starting chemotherapy in January. Can you tell me what she will experience? Does chemotherapy hurt or is it the side effects afterwards? She is in the early stage two.

Chemotherapy does not hurt. I went through chemotherapy in 2000 and didn't have any negative side affects except for hair loss. My dad didn't have any negative side affects either in 1990. But, today the treatment is more advanced and Hodgkin's has a good cure rate. I think the worst part of the Chemo is mentally thinking about it.

Epidemiology

Unlike some other lymphomas, whose incidence increases with age, Hodgkin lymphoma has a bimodal incidence curve; that is, it occurs most frequently in two separate age groups, the first being young adulthood (age 15–35) and the second being in those over 55 years old although these peaks may vary slightly with nationality.[18] Overall, it is more common in males, except for the *nodular sclerosis* variant, which is slightly more common in females. The annual incidence of Hodgkin's lymphoma is about 1 in 25,000 people, and the disease accounts for slightly less than 1% of all cancers worldwide.

The incidence of Hodgkin lymphoma is increased in patients with Human Immunodeficiency Virus infection.[19] In contrast to many other lymphomas associated with Human Immunodeficiency Virus infection it occurs most commonly in patients with higher CD4 T cell counts.

I am worried about my little girl who is 18 months old. She has at present two large lumps on her neck on either side and she has had two lumps in her head behind her right ear since she was a small baby. Is it possible that a child as young as her could have lymphoma?

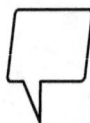

I really don't know how young a child can be to develop lymphoma. Your best bet is to ask your pediatrician, and if you're not happy, get a second opinion. Lymph glands can swell for a number of reasons, and it's not always lymphoma. They fight infection, so it could be something else.

NON-HODGKIN LYMPHOMA

The Non-Hodgkin lymphomas (NHLs) are a diverse group of hematologic cancers which encompass any lymphoma other than Hodgkin lymphoma.[1]

Lymphoma is a type of cancer derived from lymphocytes, a type of white blood cell. Many subtypes of non-Hodgkin lymphoma have been described. Non-Hodgkin lymphomas are treated by combinations of chemotherapy, monoclonal antibodies, immunotherapy, radiation, and hematopoietic stem cell transplantation.

Non-Hodgkin lymphoma are classified according to the 1982 Working Formulation, now considered obsolete. Current classifications do not separate Hodgkin from Non-Hodgkin lymphomas.

What is the maximum age of a patient diagnosed non-Hodgkin's lymphoma?

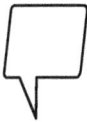

There is no maximum age, as Hodgkin's lymphoma or non-Hodgkin's can affect any age, ranging from very young children to the elderly.

History

Hodgkin's Lymphoma (HL, Hodgkin's disease), described by Thomas Hodgkin in 1832, was the first form of lymphoma described and defined. Other forms were later described and there was a need to classify them. Because Hodgkin's lymphoma was much more radiation-sensitive than other forms, its diagnosis was important for oncologists and their patients. Thus, research originally focused on it. The first classification of Hodgkin's Lymphoma was proposed by Robert J. Lukes in 1963.

While consensus was rapidly reached on the classification of Hodgkin's lymphoma, there remained a large group of very different diseases requiring further classification. The Rappaport classification, proposed by Henry Rappaport in 1956 and 1966, became the first widely accepted classification of lymphomas other than Hodgkin's. Following its publication in 1982, the Working Formulation became the standard classification for this group of diseases. It introduced the term non-Hodgkin's Lymphoma (NHL) and defined three grades of lymphoma.

However, non-Hodgkin lymphoma consists of 16 different conditions that have little in common with each other. They are grouped by their aggressiveness. Less aggressive non-Hodgkin lymphomas are compatible with a long survival while more aggressive non-Hodgkin lymphomas can be rapidly fatal without treatment. Without further narrowing, the label is of limited usefulness for patients or doctors.

The most recent lymphoma classifications, the 1994 Revised European-American Lymphoma (REAL) classification and the 2001 WHO classification, abandoned the Hodgkin lymphoma vs. non-Hodgkin lymphoma grouping. Instead, 43 different forms of lymphoma are listed and discussed separately. Although Hodgkin's lymphoma is recognized as being a tumor of lymphocytes of mature B cell lineage, it is still considered separately within the WHO classification.[2]

My friend (male, adult) got Non-Hodgkin's Lymphoma. Now he has had an unexplained consistent fever for three weeks! Doctors can't find the reason, and his body doesn't seem to be responding to the antibiotics. Any suggestion?

Does your friend have "indolent" lymphoma? With indolent lymphoma, a continuing high fever (one of the "B" symptoms) may be a sign that the cancer has transformed to a more aggressive cancer. Many patients who have had chemotherapy (CHOP plu Rituxan) at the time their non-Hodgkin lymphoma turned aggressive have had lengthy remissions--10, even 20 or more years and

*counting--especially if areas of bulky lymphoma
are irradiated.*

Modern usage of term

Nevertheless, the Working formulation and the non-Hodgkin lymphoma category continue to be used by many. To this day, lymphoma statistics are compiled as Hodgkin's vs Non-Hodgkin's lymphoma by major cancer agencies, including the National Cancer Institute in its SEER program, the Canadian Cancer Society and the IARC.

BURKITT LYMPHOMA

Burkitt lymphoma (or "Burkitt's tumor", or "Malignant lymphoma, Burkitt's type") is a cancer of the lymphatic system (in particular, B lymphocytes). It is named after Denis Parsons Burkitt, a surgeon who first described the disease in 1956 while working in equatorial Africa.

Genetics

Almost by definition, Burkitt's lymphoma is associated with c-myc gene translocation. This gene is found at 8q24.

- The most common variant is t(8;14)(q24;q32). This involves c-myc and IGH@. A variant of this, a three-way translocation, t(8;14;18), has also been identified.[3]

- A rare variant is at t(2;8)(p12;q24).[4] This involves IGK@ and c-myc.

- Another rare variant is t(8;22)(q24;q11).[4] This involves IGL@ and c-myc.

Classification

Currently Burkitt's lymphoma can be divided into three main clinical variants: the endemic, the sporadic and the immunodeficiency-associated variants.[5]

- **endemic variant** occurs in equatorial Africa. It is the most common malignancy of children in this area. Children affected with the disease often also had chronic malaria which is believed to have reduced resistance to Epstein-Barr virus (EBV) allowing it to take hold. The disease characteristically involves the jaw or other facial bone, distal ileum, cecum, ovaries, kidney or the breast.

- The **sporadic type** of Burkitt lymphoma (also known as "non-African") is another form of non-Hodgkin lymphoma found outside of Africa. The tumor cells have a similar appearance to the cancer cells of classical African or endemic Burkitt lymphoma. Again it is believed that impaired immunity provides an opening for development of the Epstein-Barr virus. Non-Hodgkins, which includes Burkitt's, accounts for 30-50% of childhood lymphoma. Jaw is less commonly involved, comparing with the endemic variant. Ileo-cecal region is the common site of involvement.

- **Immunodeficiency-associated** Burkitt lymphoma is usually associated with Human Immunodeficiency Virus infection[6] or occurs in the setting of post-transplant patients who are taking immunosuppressive drugs. Actually, Burkitt lymphoma can be the initial manifestation of AIDS.

By morphology (i.e. microscopic appearance) or immunophenotype, it is almost impossible to differentiate these three clinical variants. Immunodeficiency-associated Burkitt lymphoma may demonstrate more plasmacytic appearance or more pleomorphism, but these features are not specific.

Microscopy

Consists of sheets of monotonous (i.e. similar in size and morphology) population of medium size lymphoid cells with high proliferative activity and apoptotic activity. The "starry sky" appearance seen[7] under low power is due to scattered tingible body-laden macrophages (macrophages containing dead body of apoptotic tumor cells). The old descriptive term of "small non-cleaved cell" is misleading. The tumor cells are mostly medium in size (i.e. tumor nuclei size similar to that of histiocytes or endothelial cells). "Small non-cleaved cells" are compared to "large non-cleaved cells" of normal germinal center lymphocytes. Tumor cells possess small amount of basophilic cytoplasm. The cellular outline usually appears squared off.

Malignant B cell characteristics

Normal B cells possess rearranged immunoglobulin heavy and light chain genes, unlike most T-cells and other cells of the body in which the genes are germline. Each isolated B-cell possesses a unique IgH gene rearrangement, reminiscent of the fingerprint of a person. Since Burkitt lymphoma and other B-cell lymphomas are a clonal proliferative process, all tumor cells from one patient are supposed to possess identical IgH genes. When the DNA of tumor cells is analyzed using electrophoresis, a clonal band can be demonstrated since identical IgH genes will move to the same position. On the contrary, when a normal or reactive lymph node is analyzed using the same technique, a smear rather than a distinct band will be seen. This technique is useful since sometimes benign reactive processes (e.g. infectious mononucleosis) and malignant lymphoma can be difficult to distinguish.

Several weeks ago we were told my mother had B cell lymphoma in her bone marrow based on bone marrow biopsy results showing results that were highly suspicious. She was sent for a PET scan to see if it was any where else. Thank goodness it wasn't, but the oncologist is now saying that she doesn't have it, even though the atypical "suspicious" cells are there in her

marrow. The oncologist said we will just wait and re-test in one year, earlier if symptoms (weight loss, night sweats, fevers, swollen glands) arise. My mom lost five pounds this last week with no changes to her diet. When I asked what is significant, I never got a straight answer. She does have inconsistent night sweats (has already been through menopause), but no other symptoms. We are very confused and considering getting a second opinion. One day were told she has cancer, a couple of weeks later that she doesn't. I would appreciate any feedback you could provide.

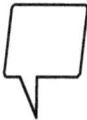

Yes, by all means get a second opinion.

Treatment

Treatment with dose-adjusted EPOCH with Rituxan (rituximab) has shown an 8 year survival rate of 91% for low risk, 90% for low-intermediate risk, 67% for high-intermediate risk, and 31% for high risk cases with few of the side effects associated with Burkitt's lymphoma chemotherapy.[8]

Effect of the chemotherapy, as with all cancers, depends on the time of diagnosis. With faster growing cancers, such as this one, the cancer actually responds faster than with slower growing cancers. This rapid response to chemotherapy can be hazardous to patient as a phenomenon called "tumor lysis syndrome" could occur. Close monitoring of patient and adequate hydration is essential during the process.

Chemotherapy

- cyclophosphamide

- doxorubicin

- vincristine

- methotrexate

- cytarabine

- ifosfamide

- etoposide

- rituximab[9]

Other treatments are immunotherapy, bone marrow transplants, surgery to remove the tumor, and radiotherapy.

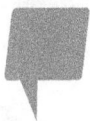

My grandmother Susie was diagnosed with Non-Hodgkin's lymphoma in 1998. She has been doing an intense herbal regime for the last

five years with good results. In September she had a mild heart attack and last week she was hospitalized for fluid in her lungs. They removed three quarts. They attribute this to the cancer. Can anyone tell me why fluid would fill the lungs, anything to help slow down this happening again, and good natural treatments for non-Hodgkin's lymphoma? Also, has anyone ever tried pancreatic enzymes for cancer? Or strong poultices?

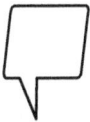

I don't have information on pancreatic enzymes, but I know someone with non-Hodgkin's who feels that Essiac Tea has helped them.

My recommendations for treating cancer:

1. See a Naturopath Doctor (they cost about the same a regular medical doctor, but insurance doesn't cover it). They will know how to change your diet, supplements and lifestyle to help become cancer free.

2. Buy organic food (including your meats) to get rid to the pesticides, hormones, antibiotics and genetically modified ingredients in your food. Pesticides have been linked to many cancers. You can find organic food at Whole Food Markets.

3. Research the Essiac Tea and decide if it's right for you.

4. Try to create a less toxic environment to help your immune system fight the cancer and not the toxins in your environment (examples: Try to use non-toxic cleaners in your home).

Epidemiology

Of all cancers involving the same class of blood cell, 2% of cases are Burkitt's lymphoma.[10]

WALDENSTRÖM'S MACROGLOBULINEMIA

Waldenström's macroglobulinemia (WM, also known as lymphoplasmacytic lymphoma) is cancer involving a subtype of white blood cells called lymphocytes. The main attributing antibody is IgM. It is a type of lymphoproliferative disease, and shares clinical characteristics with the indolent non-Hodgkin lymphomas.[1]

It is named after the Swedish physician Jan G. Waldenström, who first identified the condition.

History and classification

Waldenström's Macroglobulinemia was first described by Jan G. Waldenström (1906–1996) in 1944 in two patients with bleeding from the nose and mouth, anemia, decreased levels of fibrinogen in the blood (hypofibrinogenemia), swollen lymph nodes, neoplastic plasma cells in bone marrow, and increased viscosity of the blood due to increased levels of a class of heavy proteins called macroglobulins.[2]

For a period of time, Waldenström's Macroglobulinemia was considered to be related to multiple myeloma due to the presence of monoclonal gammopathy and infiltration of the bone marrow and other organs by plasmacytoid lymphocytes. The new World Health Organization (WHO) classification, however, places Waldenström's Macroglobulinemia under the category of lymphoplasmacytic lymphomas, itself a subcategory of the indolent (low-grade) non-Hodgkin lymphomas.[3]

Causes

Waldenstrom's macroglobulinemia is characterized by an uncontrolled clonal proliferation of terminally differentiated B lymphocytes. The underlying etiology is not yet known but a number of risk factors have been identified. There has been an association demonstrated with the locus 6p21.3 on chromosome 6.[4] There is a two- to three-fold risk increase of developing Waldenström's Macroglobulinemia in people with a personal history of autoimmune diseases with autoantibodies and particularly elevated risks associated with hepatitis, human immunodeficiency virus, and rickettsiosis.[5]

There are genetic factors, with first-degree relatives shown to have a highly increased risk of also contracting Waldenstrom's.[6]

Biochemistry

The following pathways have been implicated:

- CD154/CD40[7]

- Akt[8]

- ubiquitination, p53 activation, cytochrome c release[9]

- NF-KB[10]

- WNT/beta-catenin[11]

- mTOR[12]

- ERK[10]

- MAPK[13]

- Bcl-2[14]

Epidemiology

Of all cancers involving the same class of blood cell, 1% of cases are Waldenström's Macroglobulinemia.[15]

Waldenström's Macroglobulinemia is a rare disorder, with fewer than 1,500 cases occurring in the United States annually.[1] The median age of onset of Waldenström's Macroglobulinemia is between 60 and 65 years, with some cases occurring in late teens.[1][16]

Symptoms

Symptoms of Waldenström's Macroglobulinemia include weakness, fatigue, weight loss and chronic oozing of blood from the nose and gums.[17] Peripheral neuropathy can occur in 10% of patients. Lymphadenopathy, splenomegaly, and/or hepatomegaly are present in 30–40% of cases.[16] Some symptoms are due to the effects of the IgM paraprotein, which may cause autoimmune phenomenon or cryoglobulinemia. Other symptoms of Waldenström's Macroglobulinemia are due to the hyperviscosity syndrome, which is present in 6–20% of patients.[18][19][20][21] This is attributed to the IgM monoclonal protein increasing the viscosity of the blood. Symptoms of this are mainly neurologic and can include blurring or loss of vision.

I am a 51-year-old male that recently was sent to a hematologist because my blood labs came back abnormal. I have been running a low grade fever 99-101 for over a year and have been anemic and fatigued. Iron supplements did not help. My question is would any of the blood results point toward Lymphoma/Leukemia? I had a CT scan which showed an enlarged spleen and liver, but have no swollen lymph nodes externally. Can you have lymphoma without swollen lymph

nodes? Can lymphoma or leukemia produce low lymphocytes?

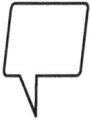

When cancer gets in the bone marrow, it grows and crowds out the normal production cells that produce normal blood cells of very kind. But low blood counts can be from other things besides cancer such as persistent infection, autoimmunity, and other things. If it were me, I'd educate myself on the basic terms so that when you sit with a doctor you can follow along.

Diagnosis

A distinguishing feature of Waldenström's Macroglobulinemia is the presence of an IgM monoclonal protein (or paraprotein) that is produced by the cancer cells.

Lab Studies

The laboratory diagnosis of Waldenström macroglobulinemia is contingent on demonstrating a significant monoclonal IgM spike and identifying malignant cells consistent with Waldenström macroglobulinemia (usually found in bone marrow biopsy samples and aspirates). General studies include a full blood count, red cell indices, platelet count, and a peripheral smear.

Normocytic normochromic anemia, leukopenia, and thrombocytopenia may be observed. Anemia is the most common finding, present in 80% of patients with symptomatic Waldenström macroglobulinemia.

The peripheral smear may reveal plasmacytoid lymphocytes, normocytic normochromic red cells, and rouleaux formation.

Neutropenia can be found in some patients.

Thrombocytopenia is found in approximately 50% of patients with bleeding diathesis. Chemistry tests include lactate dehydrogenase (LDH) levels, uric acid levels, erythrocyte sedimentation rate (ESR), renal and hepatic function, total protein levels, and an albumin-to-globulin ratio. The ESR and uric acid level may be elevated. Creatinine is occasionally elevated and electrolytes are occasionally abnormal. Hypercalcemia is noted in approximately 4% of patients. The LDH level is frequently elevated, indicating the extent of Waldenström macroglobulinemia–related tissue involvement. Rheumatoid factor, cryoglobulins, direct antiglobulin test and cold agglutinin titre results can be positive. Beta-2-microglobulin and C-reactive protein test results are not specific for Waldenström macroglobulinemia. Beta-2-

microglobulin is elevated in proportion to tumor mass. Coagulation abnormalities may be present. Prothrombin time, activated partial thromboplastin time, thrombin time, and fibrinogen tests should be performed. Platelet aggregation studies are optional. Serum protein electrophoresis results indicate evidence of a monoclonal spike but cannot establish the spike as IgM. An M component with beta-to-gamma mobility is highly suggestive of Waldenström macroglobulinemia. Immunoelectrophoresis and immunofixation studies help identify the type of immunoglobulin, the clonality of the light chain, and the monoclonality and quantitation of the paraprotein. High-resolution electrophoresis and serum and urine immunofixation are recommended to help identify and characterize the monoclonal IgM paraprotein.

The light chain of the monoclonal protein is usually the kappa light chain. At times, patients with Waldenström macroglobulinemia may exhibit more than one M protein. Plasma viscosity must be measured. Results from characterization studies of urinary immunoglobulins indicate that light chains (Bence Jones protein), usually of the kappa type, are found in the urine. Urine collections should be concentrated.

Bence Jones proteinuria is observed in approximately 40% of patients and exceeds 1 g/d in approximately 3% of patients. Patients with findings of peripheral neuropathy should have nerve conduction studies and antimyelin associated glycoprotein serology.

Prognosis

Current medical treatments result in survival of some longer than 10 years, in part this is because better diagnostic testing means early diagnosis and treatments. Older diagnosis and treatments resulted in published reports of median survival of approximately 5 years from time of diagnosis.[1] Currently, median survival is 6.5 years[22]. In rare instances, Waldenström's Macroglobulinemia progresses to multiple myeloma.[23]

The International Prognostic Scoring System for Waldenström's Macroglobulinemia (IPSSWM) is a predictive model to characterise long-term outcome.[24] According to the model, factors predicting survival are:

• age >65 years;

• hemoglobin ≤11.5 g/dL;

• platelet count ≤100×109/L;

- B2-microglobulin >3 mg/L;

- serum monoclonal protein concentration >70 g/L.

The risk categories are:

- Low: ≤1 adverse variable except age;

- Intermediate: 2 adverse characteristics or age >65 years;

- High: >2 adverse characteristics.

Five-year survival rates for these categories are 87%, 68% and 36% respectively.[25]

The International Prognostic Scoring System for Waldenstrom's Macroglobulinemia has been shown applicable to patients on a Rituximab-based treatment regimen.[25] An additional predictive factor is elevated serum lactate dehydrogenase (LDH).[26]

Treatment

There is no single accepted treatment for Waldenström's Macroglobulinemia[27]. Indeed, in 1991, Waldenström himself raised the question of the need for effective therapy.[28] In the absence of symptoms, many clinicians will recommend simply monitoring the patient[29]. Should treatment be started it should address both the paraprotein level and the lymphocytic B-cells.[30]

In 2002, a panel at the International Workshop on Waldenstrom Macroglobulinemia agreed on criteria for the initiation of therapy. They recommended starting therapy in patients with constitutional symptoms such as recurrent fever, night sweats, fatigue due to anemia, weight loss, progressive symptomatic lymphadenopathy or splenomegaly, and anemia due to marrow infiltration. Complications such as hyperviscosity syndrome, symptomatic sensorimotor peripheral neuropathy, systemic amyloidosis, renal insufficiency, or symptomatic cryoglobulinemia were also suggested as indications for therapy.[31]

Treatment includes the monoclonal antibody rituximab, sometimes in combination with chemotherapeutic drugs such as chlorambucil, cyclophosphamide, or vincristine or with thalidomide[32]. Corticosteroids may also be used in combination. Plasmapheresis can be used to treat the hyperviscosity syndrome by removing the paraprotein from the blood, although it does not address the underlying disease.[33]

Recently, autologous bone marrow transplantation has been added to the available treatment options.[34][35][36][37]

Drug pipeline

A database of clinical trials investigating Waldenstrom's macroglobulinemia is maintained by the National Institutes of Health in the US.[38]

Phase IV

• None

Phase III

• Comparison between Chlorambucil and Fludarabine[39][40]

Phase II

There are over 100 active trials studying different interventions.[41] Interventions include either individually or combinations of Fludarabine, Perifosine, Bortezomib, Rituximab, Sildenafil citrate, CC-5013, Thalidomide, Simvastatin, Campath-1H, Dexamethasone, Antineoplaston, Beta Alethine, Dolastatin 10, Cyclophosphamide, Yttrium Y 90 Ibritumomab, ABT-263, Ofatumumab, Enzastaurin and Denileukin diftitox.

PRIMARY EFFUSION LYMPHOMA

Primary effusion lymphoma (PEL) is a B-cell lymphoma

Causes

It is caused by Kaposi's sarcoma-associated herpesvirus (KSHV), also known as human herpesvirus 8 (HHV-8).[2][3]

In most cases, the lymphoma cells are also infected with Epstein Barr virus (EBV).[4]

Primary effusion lymphoma most commonly arises in patients with underlying immunodeficiency, such as AIDS.[5][6]

The condition can exist in the absence of HHV-8 and Human Immunodeficiency Virus, though this is rare.[7]

Presentation

Primary effusion lymphoma is unusual in that the majority of cases arise in body cavities, such as the pleural space or the pericardium; another name for primary effusion lymphoma is "body cavity lymphoma".

A case has been described that was positive for CD38, CD71 and CD30.[8]

History

It was recognized as a unique type of lymphoma only after the discovery of KSHV in 1994.

Prognosis

It is generally resistant to cancer chemotherapy drugs that are active against other lymphomas, and carries a poor prognosis.[9]

Sirolimus has been proposed as a treatment option.[10]

SPLENIC MARGINAL ZONE LYMPHOMA

Splenic marginal zone lymphoma (SMZL) is a lymphoma made up of B-cells that replace the normal architecture of the white pulp of the spleen. The neoplastic cells are both small lymphocytes and larger, transformed blasts, and they invade the mantle zone of splenic follicles and erode the marginal zone, ultimately invading the red pulp of the spleen. Frequently, the bone marrow and splenic hilar lymph nodes are involved along with the peripheral blood. The neoplastic cells circulating in the peripheral blood are termed villous lymphocytes due to their characteristic appearance.[1]

Synonyms

Under older classification systems, the following names were used:[1]

Classification system	Name
Rappaport	well-differentiated lymphocytic lymphoma
Lukes-Collins	small lymphocytic lymphoma
Working Formulation	small lymphocytic lymphoma
FAB	splenic lymphoma with circulating villous lymphocytes

Cause

The cell of origin is postulated to be a post-germinal center B-cell with an unknown degree of differentiation.[1]

Diagnosis

With splenic involvement a requirement for a diagnosis of splenic marginal zone lymphoma, splenomegaly is seen in almost all patients, commonly without lymphadenopathy.[1] Aside from the uniform involvement of the spleen, the bone marrow is frequently positive in patients with splenic marginal zone lymphoma. Nodal and extranodal involvement are rare.[1]

Circulating lymphoma cells are sometimes present in peripheral blood, and they occasionally show short villi at the poles of cells and plasmacytoid differentiation.[2]

Autoimmune thrombocytopenia and anemia sometimes seen in patients with splenic marginal zone lymphoma. Circulating villous lymphocytes are sometimes observed in peripheral blood samples.[1] A monoclonal paraprotein is detected in a third of patients without hypergammaglobulinemia or hyperviscosity.[3][4]

Reactive germinal centers in splenic white pulp are replaced by small neoplastic lymphocytes that efface the mantle zone and ultimately blend in with the marginal zone with occasional larger neoplastic cells that resemble blasts.[4][5] The red pulp is always involved, with both nodules of larger neoplastic cells and sheets of the small neoplastic lymphocytes. Other features that may been seen include sinus invasion, epithelial histocytes, and plasmacytic differentiation of neoplastic cells.

Involved hilar lymph nodes adjacent to the spleen show an effaced architecture without preservation of the marginal zone seen in the spleen.[1]

Splenic marginal zone lymphoma in bone marrow displays a nodular pattern with morphology similar to what is observed in the splenic hilar lymph nodes.[6]

Molecular Findings

Immunophenotype

Antigen	Status
CD20	Positive
CD79a	Positive
CD5	Negative

CD10	Negative
CD23	Negative
CD43	Negative
cyclin D1	Negative

The relevant markers that define the immunophenotype for splenic marginal zone lymphoma are shown in the table to the right.[7][8] The lack of CD5 expression is helpful in the discrimination between splenic marginal zone lymphoma and chronic lymphocytic leukemia/small lymphocytic lymphoma, and the lack of CD10 expression argues against follicular lymphoma. Mantle cell lymphoma is excluded due to the lack of CD5 and cyclin-D1 expression.[9]

Genetics

Clonal rearrangements of the immunoglobulin genes (heavy and light chains) are frequently seen.[10] The deletion 7q21-32 is seen in 40% of splenic marginal zone lymphoma patients, and translocations of the CDK6 gene located at 7q21 have also been reported.[11]

Epidemiology

Less than 1% of all lymphomas are splenic marginal zone lymphomas[12] and it is postulated that splenic marginal zone lymphoma may represent a large fraction of unclasssifiable CD5- chronic lymphocytic leukemias.[1] The typical patient is over the age of 50, and gender preference has been described

GASTRIC LYMPHOMA

Primary gastric lymphoma (lymphoma that originates in the stomach itself)[1] is an uncommon condition, accounting for less than 15% of gastric malignancies and about 2% of all lymphomas. However, the stomach is a very common extranodal site for lymphomas (lymphomas originating somewhere else with metastasis to stomach).[2] It is also the most common source of lymphomas in the gastrointestinal tract.

Clinical presentation

Primary gastric lymphoma usually affects the elderly (with peak incidence in the sixth decade of life)[4] and presenting symptoms include epigastric pain, early satiety, fatigue and weight loss.

Diagnosis

These lymphomas are often difficult to differentiate from gastric adenocarcinoma. The lesions are usually ulcers with a ragged, thickened mucosal pattern on contrast radiographs.

The diagnosis is typically made by biopsy at the time of endoscopy. Several endoscopic findings have been reported, including solitary ulcers, thickened gastric folds, mass lesions and nodules. As there may be infiltration of the submucosa, larger biopsy forceps, endoscopic ultrasound guided biopsy, endoscopic submucosal resection, or laparotomy may be required to obtain tissue.

Imaging investigations including CT scans or endoscopic ultrasound are useful to stage disease. Hematological parameters are usually checked to assist with staging and to exclude concomitant leukemia. An elevated LDH level may be suggestive of lymphoma.

Well, they ended up doing a laparotomy yesterday to remove a lymph node. I am very sore, but at least I get two weeks off of work. Won't get the results until Monday.

Are you sure you're getting the result on Monday already? Please don't be too disappointed if they don't have the result ready for you, as such things usually take time.

When I was first diagnosed, I was told two weeks after I had my biopsy that it was lymphoma - but had to wait another week or two to get a certain answer about which lymphoma type. 15 days ago I also had a laparoscopy to remove a lymph node in my abdomen, as they believe I have relapsed. They told me the result would be back in two-three weeks. I called the hospital two days ago to check, but it was still not ready, so they told me to call again in another week. I don't want to make you more frustrated; I'm just thinking you should be prepared that it MIGHT take longer so you won't be too disappointed on Monday.

I have been concerned about a mass in my neck and nodes behind my ear that have been swollen for eight weeks. I got checked today and my doctor wasn't concerned about the places I thought were trouble. He found a node on the right side of my neck that he said he wasn't "overly concerned" with but wanted me to do a CT scan Friday. At that point they may draw some fluid from it to do a biopsy.

I'm going though the same thing. All I can say is it's a process. I've had three scans and two biopsies, been on antibiotics two times to see if they would shrink. My biopsies came back non-carcinoma. Also usually they get bigger if there is a problem.

The doctor can sense that you are scared and he is being proactive. I have a swollen neck lymph node *too. The ultrasound showed that it looked normal. The fine needle biopsy failed and only drew out blood. The next step is an ultrasound guided biopsy.*

Histopathology

The majority of gastric lymphomas are non-Hodgkin's lymphoma of B-cell origin. These tumors may range from well-differentiated, superficial involvements (MALT) to high-grade, large-cell lymphomas.

Other lymphomas involving the stomach include mantle cell lymphoma and T-cell lymphomas which may be associated with enteropathy; the latter usually occur in the small bowel but have been reported in the stomach.

Risk factors

Risk factors for gastric lymphoma include the following:

• *Helicobacter pylori*[5]

• Long-term immunosuppressant drug therapy

• Human Immunodeficiency Virus infection

Treatment

Diffuse large B-cell lymphomas of the stomach are primarily treated with chemotherapy with CHOP with or without rituximab being a usual first choice.

Antibiotic treatment to eradicate H. pylori is indicated as first line therapy for MALT lymphomas. About 60% of MALT lymphomas completely regress with eradication therapy[6]. Second line therapy for MALT lymphomas is usually chemotherapy with a single agent, and complete response rates of greater than 70% have gain been reported[7].

Subtotal gastrectomy, with post-operative chemotherapy is undertaken in refractory cases, or in the setting of complications, including gastric outlet obstruction.

> *My husband has only had two CHOP treatments, and then all of a sudden he had severe pain on the left side of his face and head. The oncologist knew exactly what is was: shingles! He's now on a large does of Valtrex and good pain medication. CHOP is stopped for now. Anyone else have this happen? How long until you can start treatment again?*

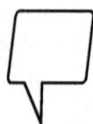

My dad has follicular lymphoma and developed shingles on one arm. His symptoms lasted about two weeks. The rash was extremely red and very blotchy looking. He was diagnosed by a dermatologist. He is fine now, except that they can't find a chemotherapy that works and his stomach is quite distended from the lymph fluid. He has had two parathensitis procedures, but to no avail.

FOLLICULAR LYMPHOMA

Follicular lymphoma is the second most common of the indolent non-Hodgkin's lymphomas. It is defined as a lymphoma of follicle center B-cells (centrocytes and centroblasts), which has at least a partially follicular pattern. It is positive for CD10,[1] and usually negative for CD5.[2]

There are several synonymous and obsolete terms for this disease, such as CB/CC lymphoma (Centroblastic and Centrocytic lymphoma), nodular lymphoma[3] and Brill-Symmers Disease.

I was diagnosed last week with stage III or IV non-Hodgkin's follicular lymphoma. I'll have a bone marrow biopsy next week and a port installed to start chemotherapy. My doctor wants to do chemotherapy first (R-CHOP), then try to get in a clinical trial in which they follow chemotherapy with radio-immunotherapy, then a stem cell transplant. Is anybody in this situation?

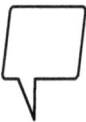

I have recently finished my chemotherapy for follicular non-Hodgkin's lymphoma, and I am healthy again. My port was taken out and my life is back to normal. Hang in there; your life will be brighter and better when you are done.

Morphology

The tumor is composed of follicles containing a mixture of centrocytes (WHO nomenclature) or cleaved follicle center cells (older American nomenclature), "small cells", and centroblasts (WHO nomenclature) or large noncleaved follicle center cells (older American nomenclature), "large cells". These follicles are surrounded by non-malignant cells, mostly T-cells. In the follicles, centrocytes typically predominate; centroblasts are usually in minority.

I am a 39-year-old female. I was diagnosed today with B cell follicular lymphoma, but have not been given the stage yet after my biopsy. My PET scan report says that "there is a huge mass occupying the right lung with direct invasion of the mediastinum and hilum. This mass measures 11.4 x 8.7 cm with the maximum SUV of 16.16. There are two small adjacent pulmonary masses extending into the lower lobe, each at approximately 3cm. Maximum SUV 9.17. There is diffuse abnormal interstitial lung disease. I do not appreciate evidence to suggest distant metastatic disease." Has anyone else had it present in this way? I am under the impression

they need to get the large one under control rather quickly as I can't breathe.

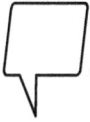

Many people who have large tumors notice an extreme shrinkage after the first treatment, so that may offer you some relief in the breathing department.

Grading

According to the WHO criteria, the disease is morphologically graded into:[4]

• grade 1 (<5 centroblasts per high-power field (hpf))

• grade 2 (6–15 centroblasts/hpf)

• grade 3 (>15 centroblasts/hpf).

Grade 3 is further subdivided into:

• grade 3a (centrocytes still present)

• the rare grade 3b (the follicles consist almost entirely of centroblasts)

The clinical relevance of this grading system is debated, although grades 1, 2 and 3a can be treated as an indolent disease, while grade 3b is an aggressive disease. Occasional cases may show plasmacytoid differentiation or foci of marginal zone or monocytoid B-cells.

> *How long can you live with stage 4 follicular lymphoma without any difficulty?*

> *With several possible treatment plans, there is no reason why you cannot live for several years, but everyone is different and there are no certainties in life. It is important to get regular checkups so any possible recurrences can be caught early and either treated if appropriate or watched carefully.*

Causes

A translocation between chromosome14 and 18 results in the overexpression of the bcl-2 gene.[5] As the bcl-2 protein is normally involved in preventing apoptosis, cells with an overexpression of this protein are basically immortal. The bcl-2 gene is normally found on chromosome 18, and the translocation moves the gene near to the site of the immunoglobulin heavy chain enhancer element on chromosome 14.

Translocations of BCL6 at 3q27 can also be involved.[6]

> *I am 40 years old and diagnosed with follicular lymphoma stage 1 last January. I had Rituxan treatments in October and go back in July for another CT and possibly treatments again. I am curious how many of you have this cancer,*

how long you have had it, and what types of treatments you have had.

I have had follicular lymphoma for a little under 11 years. I also was diagnosed at about your age. While it is not usually considered curable, I think you will find that there is a great deal of reason to hope for a cure at only Stage I. Radiation alone can sometimes cure it that early. But even at Stage IV like I was, you will find it is a very manageable disease.

I was diagnosed in July 2006 with Stage IV Grade 1 indolent follicular lymphoma and was treated with Fludarabine (x4) Cytoxan (x3) and Rituxan (x6) and had a complete clinical remission, i.e. nodes in mesentery became miniscule. Since then I have annual scans. Feel great and hoping my next scan in late August does not show any recurrence. It is certainly a manageable form of lymphoma.

Treatment

There is no consensus regarding the best treatment algorithm, but watch-and-wait policies, (combinations of) alkylators and nucleoside analogues, anthracycline-containing regimens (eg. CHOP), rituximab, autologous and allogeneic hematopoietic stem cell transplantation have all been applied. The disease is regarded as incurable (although allogeneic stem cell transplanation may be curative, the mortality from the procedure is too high to be a first line option). The exception is localized disease, which can be cured by local irradiation. The typical pattern is one of good responses from treatment, followed by relapses some years later.

I got my results back yesterday. It is follicular lymphoma. I am getting a bone marrow biopsy done on Friday. I have decided to wait and watch on my treatment. With it being a slow growing cancer, and I have no B symptoms yet, I have made the decision (along with the oncologist) to wait and have another CT scan done in August. Everyone thinks I am crazy for just waiting to see what happens. What do you think? I feel I have read everything there is to read on follicular lymphoma, and I am pretty confident in my decision.

The best thing that you can do is stay positive and listen to your doctor. I don't think that he (or she) would recommend that course of action if it wasn't appropriate for you.

Prognosis

Median survival is around 10 years, but the range is wide, from less than one year, to more than 20 years. Some patients may never need treatment.

> *Four years ago today I got that call saying I had follicular Non-Hodgkin's Lymphoma. In the beginning of my journey, I was afraid of all the things I would miss, especially the milestones of my children's lives. At some point along the road, I learned to live to live, not live in fear of dying.*

Epidemiology

Of all cancers involving the same class of blood cell, 22% of cases are follicular lymphomas.

> *Is follicular lymphoma common in teens?*

No, it is not.

ANAPLASTIC LARGE CELL LYMPHOMA

Anaplastic large cell lymphoma (ALCL) is a type of non-Hodgkin lymphoma that features in the World Health Organization (WHO) classification of lymphomas.

Its name derives from anaplasia and large cell lymphoma.

Signs and symptoms

It occurs in both nodal and extranodal locations. It typically presents at a late stage and is often associated with systemic symptoms ("B symptoms"). Granulomas may be present.[1]

> *I have several lumps in neck. My blood tests were all normal. During the ultrasound, they found something on the left side of neck. Before the biopsy, the radiologist said that he would wait to do biopsy and do another ultrasound in a few months. But I was already there, in the gown, the deductible paid for, so I told him to do it. The biopsy was inconclusive, and they recommended removal. I asked my family doctor about waiting and he said quite clearly, "I would get it removed." How much can they really tell from an ultrasound?*

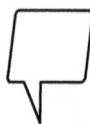

You can't tell much from an ultrasound. If a person has lymphoma, having it surgically removed doesn't change much. The lymphoma cells have been moving around anyway. Resection is for alleviating any problems that a particular tumor causes, say like blocking the throat (but then you balance the danger of surgery at a spot like inside the throat and might decide against). You do have a right to any report on any scan or test that was done.

Diagnosis

To make this diagnosis under its present system of classification, the WHO the presence of "hallmark" cells and immunopositivity for CD30.

The classification acknowledges as typical, but does not require, immunopositivity for ALK (anaplastic lymphoma kinase) protein. It specifically excludes primary cutaneous T-cell lymphomas and other specific types of anaplastic lymphoma (particularly those of B-cell lineage) with CD30 positivity.

The hallmark cells are of medium size and feature abundant cytoplasm (which may be clear, amphophilic or eosinophilic), kidney shaped nuclei, and a paranuclear eosinophilic region. Occasional cells may be identified in which the plane of section passes through the nucleus in such a way that it appears to enclose a region of cytoplasm within a ring; such cells are called "doughnut" cells.

By definition, on histological examination, hallmark cells are always present. Where they are not present in large numbers, they are usually located around blood vessels. Morphologic variants include the following types:

- Common (featuring a predominance of hallmark cells)

- Small cell (featuring smaller cells with the same immunophenotype as the hallmark cells)

- Lymphohistiocytic

- Sarcomatoid

- Signet ring

My doctor sent me for a chest x-ray, which came back clear, so he wished to proceed with no further investigation. It has now been another two months, and I still have the lumps! At present I have one on my left jaw (smaller than a pea), three on my left side of neck (pea sized), and one under left armpit (baked bean sized). I went back to a different doctor yesterday, who is now going to refer me to a specialist.

I had similar problems with a lymph node in my neck before. The lymph node swelled up to roughly the size of a ping-pong ball. I had it for about three months. I also didn't really have any other symptoms. My doctor told me it was likely due to my body fighting off a viral infection, but to be safe my doctor put me on some antibiotics. I recovered from it with no problems. It sounds like this could be the same case for you.

Have they discussed with you at all that you may just have an infection? I would suggest it. Lymph nodes are your body's normal response to infection; if you have a few swollen, that is probably the case. I've had my lymph nodes swell up to rather impressive sizes before and it was never anything serious. Usually it was just my body fighting off a viral infection or I found out I had a cut or something that was a bit infected and my body was fighting it.

Ask your Doctor for an ESR blood test. That measures whether you could be fighting some infection in your body without realizing it; usually *if that comes back higher than normal they will do further investigations.*

Immunophenotype

The hallmark cells (and variants) show immunopositivity for CD30[2][3] (also known as Ki-1). True positivity requires localisation of signal to the cell membrane and/or paranuclear region (cyptolasmic positivity is considered non-specific and non-informative). Another useful marker which helps to differentiate this lesion from Hodgkin lymphoma is Clusterin. The neoplastic cells have a golgi staining pattern (hence paranuclear staining), which is characteristic of this lymphoma. The cells are also typically positive for a subset of markers of T-cell lineage. However, as with other T-cell lymphomas, they are usually negative for the pan T-cell marker CD3. Occasional examples are of null (neither T nor B) cell type. These lymphomas show immunopositivity for anaplastic lymphoma kinase protein in 70% of cases. They are also typically positive for EMA. In contrast to many B-cell anaplastic CD30 positive lymphomas, they are negative for markers of Epstein-Barr Virus (EBV).

Molecular biology

The majority of cases, greater than 90%, contain a clonal rearrangement of the T-cell receptor. This may be identified using PCR techniques, such as T-gamma multiplex PCR. Oncogeneic potential is conferred by upregulation of a tyrosine kinase gene on chromosome 2. Several different translocations involving this gene have been identified in different cases of this lymphoma. The most common is a chromosomal translocation involving the nucleophosmin gene on chromosome 5. The translocation may be identified by analysis of giemsa-banded metaphase spreads of tumour cells and is characterised by t(2;5)(p23;q35). The product of this fusion gene may be identified by immunohistochemistry using antiserum to anaplastic lymphoma kinase protein. Probes are available to identify the translocation by fluorescent in situ hybridization. The nucleophosmin component associated with the commonest translocation results in nuclear positivity as well as cytoplasmic positivity. Positivity with the other translocations may be confined to the cytoplasm.

Differential diagnosis and diagnostic pitfalls

As the appearance of the hallmark cells, pattern of growth (nesting within lymph nodes) and positivity for EMA may mimic metastatic carcinoma, it is important to include markers for cytokeratin in any diagnostic panel (these will be negative in the case of anaplastic lymphoma). Other mimics include CD30 positive B-cell lymphomas with anaplastic cells (including Hodgkin lymphomas). These are identified by their positivity for markers of B-cell lineage and frequent presence of markers of EBV. Primary cutaneous T-cell lymphomas may also be positive for CD30; these are excluded by their anatomic distribution. anaplastic lymphoma kinase positivity may also be seen in some large cell B-cell lymphomas and occasionally in rhabdomyosarcomas.

Treatment

• Managed under "Aggressive Lymphoma" guidelines

  • CHOP is first line of treatment, CHOP-Rituxan in the unlikely scenario that CD20 is positive, given that CD20 is a B-cell marker.

  • Radiation therapy as per institutional preference (based on ECOG, SWOG, and GELA trials), but usually added for bulky disease

- Overall better prognosis than other "Aggressive Lymphomas"

  - anaplastic lymphoma kinase+ 5-year survival 70–80%

  - anaplastic lymphoma kinase- 5-year survival 30–50%

Prognosis

During treatment, relapses may occur but these typically remain sensitive to chemotherapy.

Those with anaplastic lymphoma kinase positivity have a better prognosis. It is possible that anaplastic lymphoma kinase-negative anaplastic large cell lymphomas represent other T-cell lymphomas that are morphologic mimics of anaplastic large cell lymphoma in a final common pathway of disease progression. It is possible that existing systems of classification will be revised in the future to exclude such lymphomas from this specific diagnosis.

How long can a person live with T-cell lymphoma if they do not take treatments?

It all depends on how fast the disease spreads. Please know that nobody can give you a definite answer. I also would encourage you to get informed on treatments, as they have come a long way. Yes there are several downsides, but they can save your life. Please contact the lymphoma and leukemia society in your area. They are there to help.

Epidemiology

The lymphoma is more common in the young and in males.

A 2008 study found an increased risk of anaplastic large cell lymphoma of the breast in women with silicone breast implants, although the overall risk remained exceedingly low due to the rare occurrence of the tumor.[4]

PRIMARY CNS LYMPHOMA

A primary CNS lymphoma (PCNSL) is a primary intracranial tumor appearing primarily in patients with severe immunosuppression (typically patients with AIDS). Primary CNS lymphomas represent around 20% of all cases of lymphomas in Human Immunodeficiency Virus infections (other types are Burkitt's lymphomas and immunoblastic lymphomas). Primary CNS lymphoma is highly associated with Epstein-Barr virus (EBV) infection (>90%) in immunodeficient patients (such as those with AIDS and those iatrogenically immunosuppressed)[1], and does not have a predilection for any particular age group. Mean CD4+ count at time of diagnosis is ~50/uL. Because of the severity of immunosuppression at the time of diagnosis, it is no surprise that prognosis is usually poor. In immunocompetent patients (that is, patients who do not have AIDS or some other immunodeficiency), there is rarely an association with EBV infection or other DNA viruses. In the immunocompetent population, primary CNS lymphomas typically appear in older patients in their 50's and 60's. Importantly, the incidence of primary CNS lymphoma in the immunocompetent population has been reported to have increased more than 10-fold from 2.5 cases to 30 cases per 10 million population[2][3]. The cause for the increase in incidence of this disease in the immunocompetent population is unknown.

What is "CNS lymphoma?"

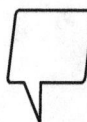

CNS lymphoma is when the disease is in the central nervous system. It can be either primary, when it starts there, or secondary, when it has started somewhere else and spread. Hodgkin's, both classical and lymphocyte predominant very rarely spreads to the brain, although cases have been reported. Virtually all cases are diffuse b-cell lymphomas, which is an aggressive form of non-Hodgkin's lymphoma. Unfortunately classical Hodgkin's and particularly lymphocyte predominant can transform to diffuse b-cell lymphoma.

Classification

Most primary CNS lymphomas are diffuse large B cell non-Hodgkin lymphomas[4][5].

Clinical manifestations

A primary CNS lymphoma usually presents with seizure, headache, cranial nerve findings, altered mental status, or other focal neurological deficits typical of a mass effect[6][7]. Systemic symptoms may include fever, night sweats, or weight loss.

What else can cause chronic swollen lymph nodes besides cancer?

Generalized lymphadenopathy can be associated with a number of chronic infections or blood disorders. What you want to find out is: are there other symptoms together with the swellings? For example: pain, fever, tiredness, nausea, headaches, weight loss, anything at all. Sometimes people pick up a mild infection and become carriers of the disease (bacteria or virus) or parasite; they may have swollen lymph glands but nothing else shows. I would make a timeline of when you first noticed the swellings, where you noticed them first, and where did they spread to first. Then ask yourself about other medical complaints you may have had since then. Those problems that are recurrent are more important. Those that happen frequently may be linked to the

*swellings. Best advice would be to have yourself
examined by a doctor.*

Diagnosis

MRI or contrast enhanced CT usually shows multiple
(one to three) 3 to 5 cm ring-enhancing lesions in
almost any location, but usually deep in the white
matter. The major differential diagnosis is cerebral
toxoplasmosis, which is also prevalent in AIDS
patients and also presents with a ring-enhanced
lesion, although toxoplasmosis generally presents
with more lesions and the contrast enhancement is
more pronounced.

Because imaging techniques cannot distinguish
the two conditions with certainty, patients usually
undergo a brain biopsy if the lesion is solitary or if a
trial of toxoplasmosis therapy is non-therapeutic. In
the future, it may be possible to use a PCR assay of
cerebrospinal fluid for EBV DNA.

*I'm a 17-year-old male. I've been worried that
I have lymphoma for five years. My lymph
nodes in the neck and groin have been slightly
swollen throughout this time period. Recently
I've gone to the doctor to have multiple blood
tests, an ultrasound, and a CT scan. My blood
tests show elevated bilirubin, but my CT scan*

shows nothing around my liver or bile duct. They suspect Gilbert's syndrome. The ultrasound showed lymph nodes around the pancreas, with the largest being 2cms long. I have an increased awareness of anything that might point to bad health: slightly ridged finger and toe nails, brittle hair that falls out easily (no noticeable hair loss), dry skin and hair, new moles and bumps on my skin, and my health obsessed mindset. What can I do to assure myself that I'm not sick?

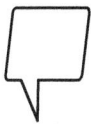

I would think if you've been thinking you've had lymphoma for five years, you would have more symptoms present such as weight loss, fatigue, itchy skin, night sweats, etc. To clear your mind, make a doctor's appointment and mention possible lymphoma to your doctor.

Treatment

Surgical resection is usually ineffective because of the depth of the tumor. Treatment with irradiation and corticosteroids often only produces a partial response, but tumor recurs in more than 90% of patients. Median survival is 10–18 months in immunocompetent patients, and less in those with AIDS. The addition of IV methotrexate and citrovorum may extend survival to a median of 3.5 years. If radiation is added to methotrexate, median survival time may increase beyond four years. However, radiation is not recommended in conjunction with methotrexate because of an increased risk of leukoencephalopathy and dementia in patients older than 60.[8] In AIDS patients, perhaps the most important factor with respect to treatment is the use of highly active anti-retroviral therapy (HAART), which affects the CD4+ lymphocyte population and the level of immunosuppression.

MANTLE CELL LYMPHOMA

Mantle cell lymphoma (MCL) is one of the rarer of the non-Hodgkin's lymphomas (NHLs), comprising about 6% of non-Hodgkin lymphoma cases.[1] There are only about 15,000 patients presently in the U.S. (The prevalence seems to be somewhat higher in Europe.) While it is difficult to treat and seldom considered cured, investigations into better treatments are actively pursued worldwide. Median survival times were about three years, but are now estimated as approaching six years for new patients.

Mantle cell lymphoma is a subtype of B-cell lymphoma, due to CD5 positive antigen-naive pregerminal center B-cell within the mantle zone that surrounds normal germinal center follicles. Mantle cell lymphoma cells generally over-express cyclin D1 due to a **t(11:14)**[2] chromosomal translocation in the DNA. More specifically, the translocation is at t(11;14)(q13;q32).[3][4]

The cause is unknown and not genetic. Mantle cell lymphoma is not communicable. It essentially is an abnormal break and subsequent translocation in a gene that causes the cells to divide too early before becoming capable of helping to fight diseases. In addition, the cells do not die as they should and therefore accumulate in the lymphoid system, including lymph nodes and the spleen, with non-useful cells eventually rendering the system dysfunctional. Mantle cell lymphoma affected cells proliferate in a *nodular* or *diffuse* pattern with two main cytologic variants: *typical* or *blastic*. Typical cases are small to intermediate sized cells with irregular nuclei. Blastic (aka *blastoid*) variants have intermediate to large sized cells with finely dispersed chromatin and are more aggressive in nature.[5]

Symptoms

The ratio of males to females affected is about 4:1. At diagnosis, the typical patient is in their 60s and usually presents to the oncologist with advanced disease. About half have either fever, heavy night sweats, unexplained weight loss (over 10%) or some combination. Swelling of lymph nodes and spleen are usually present. Bone marrow, liver and GI tract involvement occurs in a very high percentage.

It is common for a person to have initially noticed "a bump" on the neck or in the armpits or groin.

I've got a sort of vexing issue that's plagued me for a good 18 months. Multiple doctors and dentists haven't been able to figure it out; in fact, no one can say for sure if its the problem

is dental or more of an HENT issue. I have mild inflammation in and around the right lower-rear part of my mouth, right where my wisdom tooth was pulled from a good 15+ years ago. It stretches to the point where my gums meet my cheek. My dentists have said they don't see anything. I took some antibiotics once, and it seemed to help a bit, but then just came back to normal after about two weeks.

After six months ago, I noticed that two of my submandibular lymph nodes were swollen. They aren't huge, maybe 1 cm or 1.5 cm. They don't really hurt, and I still have them to this day, which of course makes me concerned about lymphoma. I swear that when I push on them, I feel a reaction in my swollen gums! It seems associated.

A general practitioner has recently checked out the swollen nodes and said they were insignificant - too small and not very hard. Any thoughts or theories appreciated!

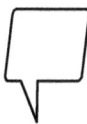

I would suggest a follow-up with an Ear/Nose/Throat specialist. My husband is currently recovering from oral cancer treatments - base of tongue cancer. His ONLY symptom was a pain free lump in his neck which he thought was a swollen gland. It turned out to be a malignant lymph node.

About two months ago I noticed that a lymph node in my neck was swollen. I didn't feel bad or anything; I figured I must be trying to develop some type of infection. About two weeks later I began to stay really tired all the time. I also noticed another swollen node directly below the original. I let that go as well. I now have a total of seven swollen lumps in my neck and one just to the right of my collarbone. I am constantly tired and my feet and neck itch like crazy, especially at night. Should I be concerned about lymphoma? What could be another cause for this swelling?

You should get to a doctor. A simple blood test will tell you most everything usually.

Diagnosis

Diagnosis generally requires stained slides of a surgically removed part of a lymph node. Other methods are also commonly used, including cytogenetics and fluorescence in situ hybridization (FISH). Polymerase chain reaction (PCR) and CER3 clonotypic primers are additional methods, but are less often used.

The immunophenotype profile consists of CD5+ (in about 80%)[6], CD10-/+,It is usually CD5+ and CD10-.[7] CD20+, CD23-/+ (though plus in rare cases). Generally cyclin D1 is expressed but it may not be required. The workup for Mantle cell lymphoma is similar to the workup for many indolent lymphomas and certain aggressive lymphomas.

Mantle cell lymphoma is a systemic disease with frequent involvement of the bone marrow and gastrointestinal tract (generally showing polyposis in the lining). There is also a not-uncommon leukemic phase, marked by presence in the blood. For this reason, both the peripheral blood and bone marrow are evaluated for the presence of malignant cells. Chest, abdominal, and pelvic CT scans are routinely performed.

Since mantle cell lymphoma may present a lymphomatous polyposis coli and colon involvement is common, colonoscopy is now considered a routine part of the evaluation. Upper endoscopy and neck CT scan may be helpful in selected cases. In some patients with the blastic variant, lumbar puncture is done to evaluate the spinal fluid for involvement.

I have a healthy 16-year-old son who a month ago started a dry cough and feeling fatigued; on the back of his neck he has a small raised lymph node. I assumed he had a possible allergy thing going on and treated him with over the counter medications. It has now been a month since the onset of symptoms and now he has several large (over an inch) lymph nodes in his groin area and several smaller ones in his neck. I took him to the doctors she ordered a CT of his abdomen and pelvis. The original findings showed a high density mass in his chest wall where the CT cut off. My son goes today for an ultrasound of the largest of the nodes (right hip/groin area). I cant help but feel there is something very wrong with my son and I feel like his doctor isn't considering anything other than a "mono type illness" - what does this mean? Can your blood, urine and CT be normal but this be cancer, or is my doctor right?

If your son's blood test results come back normal it does not mean he does not have cancer. His symptoms can definitely be a cause of many things, but they are a cause for concern. Please insist on a biopsy; it is a quick procedure that will provide you with the answers you need. Lymph nodes will swell up if he's running an infection.

Causes

Attempts to determine causes of mantle cell lymphoma have failed. It is not known what causes the translocation damage to the gene. Exposure to toxins is often mentioned as a possibility. The translocation damage to a gene is required in only one cell for the cancer to begin.

Prognosis

Prognosis of mantle cell lymphoma is problematic and indexes do not work as well due to patients presenting with advanced stage disease. Staging is used but is not very informative, since the malignant B-cells can travel freely though the lymphatic system and therefore most patients are at stage II or IV at diagnosis. Prognosis is not strongly affected by staging in mantle cell lymphoma and the concept of metastasis does not really apply.

The Mantle Cell Lymphoma International Prognostic Index (MIPI) was derived from a data set of 455 advanced stage mantle cell lymphoma patients treated in series of clinical trials in Germany/Europe. Of the evaluable population, approximately 18% were treated with high-dose therapy and stem cell transplantation in first remission. The MIPI is able to classify patients into three risk groups: low risk (median survival not reached after median 32 mos follow-up and 5-year OS rate of 60%), intermediate risk (median survival 51 months) and high risk (median survival 29 months). In addition to the four independent prognostic factors included in the model, the cell proliferation index (Ki-67) was also shown to have additional prognostic relevance. When the Ki67 is available, a biologic MIPI can be calculated.[8]

(The letter A after the Roman numeral indicates that normal external symptoms are not present. The Letter B indicates the symptoms are present and hence they are called "B Symptoms".)

Mantle cell lymphoma is one of the few non-Hodgkin lymphomas that can cross the boundary into the brain, yet it can be treated in that event.

There are a number of prognostic indicators that have been studied. There is not universal agreement on their importance or usefulness in prognosis.

Ki-67 is an indicator of how fast cells mature and is expressed in a range from about 10% to 90%. The lower the percentage, the lower the speed of maturity, and the more indolent the disease. Katzenberger et al. Blood 2006;107:3407 graphs survival versus time for subsets of patients with varying Ki-67 indices. He shows median survival times of about one year for 61–90% Ki-67 and nearly four years for 5–20% Ki-67 index.

Mantle cell lymphoma cell types can aid in prognosis in a subjective way. Blastic is a larger cell type. Diffuse is spread through the node. Nodular are small groups of collected cells spread through the node. Diffuse and nodular are similar in behavior. Blastic is faster growing and it is harder to get long remissions. Some thought is that given a long time, some non-blastic mantle cell lymphoma transforms to blastic. Although survival of most blastic patients is shorter, some data shows that 25% of blastic mantle cell lymphoma patients survive to five years. That is longer than diffuse type and almost as long as nodular (almost seven years).

Beta-2 microglobulin is another risk factor in mantle cell lymphoma used primarily for transplant patients. Values less than three have yielded 95% overall survival to six years for auto SCT where over three yields a median of 44 months overall survival for auto SCT (Khouri 03). This is not yet fully validated.

Testing for high levels of LDH in non-Hodgkin lymphoma patients is useful because LDH is released when body tissues break down for *any* reason. While it cannot be used as a sole means of diagnosing non-Hodgkin lymphoma, it is a surrogate for tracking tumor burden in those diagnosed by other means. The normal range is approximately 100–190.

Key diagnostics for mantle cell lymphoma

- CT Scan - Computerized tomography scan yields images of part or whole body. Gives a large number of slices on X-ray image.

- PET Scan - Generally of the whole body, shows a three-dimensional image of where previously injected radioactive glucose is metabolized at a rapid rate. Faster-than-average metabolism shows as a black area and indicates that cancer is likely present. Metabolism of radioactive glucose may give a false positive, particularly if the patient has exercised before the test.

PET scans are much more effective when the information from them is integrated with that from a CT scan to show more precisely where the cancer activity is located and to more accurately measure the size of tumors.

I am pleased to report that my last PET scan returned a normal study. Absolutely no traces of my stage IIIa NS Hodgkin's. So I am now a

couple of treatments away from getting back to a slightly revised lifestyle. Due to some low neutrophil counts early in the ABVD regimen, I was off put back into the following week and off schedule. Well, I think my oncologist got a little confused on where exactly I was in the schedule and ordered my PET in the middle of the fourth cycle instead of at the end of it, effectively reaching this positive conclusion a half cycle early. I have done my homework over these last months and one recurring rule of thumb presented is that treatment should extend two cycles beyond a negative scan. If this is the case, it would stand to reason that treatment should end one treatment early. Now I fully understand that one more treatment isn't that big of a deal in the scheme of things and a PET scan isn't a guarantee of anything. I am however, a scientist and curious if there is any precedent out there of people ending ABVD early be it a half cycle or otherwise.

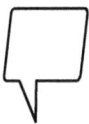

I had a scan 2/3 of the way through six cycles of ABVD, and continued until all 12 treatments were complete. I'd rather err on the side of a bit too much ABVD, than not enough. I'll take my chances with the long term side effects in place of a possible relapse

I received a no trace report also after my second cycle. It was recommended that I continue and complete the process. I wanted to stop, but I know that it would give my family more comfort knowing that the cycle was completed. I finished it with little to no side effects. I would complete the cycle to make sure.

About a year ago I noticed a small fixed lump in the back of my neck. I went to the general practitioner and was told to monitor it. A couple of months later, I discovered another few lumps in my neck (these were moveable) and noticed that my lymph nodes in my groin on both sides were enlarged. I decided to go back to a different general practitioner and was referred. I had lots of blood tests done and a CT scan, both of which came back clear. Is there any way that I could still have anything nasty if both showed the all clear?

I would definitely keep pushing the doctors. I would give the doctor a call and clarify what he said, because if your lymph nodes were swollen at the time, they would definitely show up on the CT scan. A common practice is to order the CT scan

*with and without contrast, along with a PET scan
and blood work. That is the most comprehensive
way to test for Lymphoma. Also, Lymphomas are
most responsive to treatments when they are in
their active stage (growing quickly). So if it is a
slow growing type of Lymphoma, the doctors will
wait to treat it until it starts growing quickly. Many
cancers can be diagnosed with blood tests alone,
but with Lymphoma, this is not the case.*

*I had a lymphoma about the size of a grapefruit
on my abdominal wall. After four rounds of
chemotherapy, my PET scan showed no signs of
lymphoma. How reliable is the PET scan, and
should I continue my treatments if there is no sign
of cancer?*

*A PET scan is usually pretty reliable. But, the fact
that people relapse after periods of remission
shows that lymphoma cells can remain which were
not possible to detect.*

Treatments

There are no proven standards of treatment for
mantle cell lymphoma, and not even consensus
among specialists on how to treat it optimally.
Many regimens are available and often get good

response rates, but patients almost always get disease progression after chemotherapy. Each relapse is typically more difficult to treat, and relapse is generally faster. Fortunately, regimens are available that will treat relapse, and new approaches are under test. Because of the aforementioned factors, many mantle cell lymphoma patients enroll in clinical trials to get the latest treatments.

There are four classes of treatments currently in general use: chemotherapy, immune based therapy, radioimmunotherapy and new biologic agents. The phases of treatment are generally: frontline, following diagnosis, consolidation, after frontline response (to prolong remissions), and relapse. Relapse is usually experienced multiple times.

Chemotherapy

Chemotherapy is widely used as frontline treatment, and often is not repeated in relapse due to side effects. Alternate chemotherapy is sometimes used at first relapse. For frontline treatment, CHOP with rituximab (Rituxan, Mabthera) is the most common chemotherapy, and often given as outpatient by IV. A stronger chemotherapy with greater side effects (mostly hematologic) is HyperCVAD, often given as in-patient, with rituximab and generally to fitter

patients (some of which are over 65). HyperCVAD is becoming popular and showing promising results, especially with rituximab. It can be used on some elderly (over 65) patients, but seems only beneficial when the baseline Beta-2-MG blood test was normal. It is showing better complete remissions (CR) and progression free survival (PFS) than CHOP regimens. Another chemotherapy class is fludarabine monotherapy, sometimes combined with cyclophosphamide and mitoxatrone, usually with rituximab. Cladribine and clofarabine are two other drugs being investigated in mantle cell lymphoma. Cytotoxic chemotherapies, including bendamustin, are being studied alone and with similar combinations. A relatively new regimen that uses old drugs is PEP-C, which includes relatively small, daily doses of prednisone, etoposide, procarbazine, and cyclophosphamide, taken orally, has proven effective for relapsed patients. According to John Leonard M.D., a key researcher/proponent of PEP-C, may have anti-angiogenetic properties[3][4], something that he and his colleagues are testing through an ongoing drug trial[5].

Another approach involves using very high doses of chemotherapy, sometimes combined with total body irradiation (TBI), in an attempt to destroy all evidence of the disease. The downside to this is the destruction of the patients' entire immune system as well, requiring rescue by transplantation of a new immune system (Hematopoietic stem cell transplantation), using either ones' own previously treated and stored stem cells (an autologous stem cell transplant), or those from a matched donor (an allogeneic stem cell transplant). A presentation at the December 2007 American Society of Hematology (ASH) conference by Christian Geisler, chairman of the Nordic Lymphoma Group [6] (Copenhagen, Denmark), claimed that according to trial results, mantle cell lymphoma is potentially curable with very intensive chemo-immunotherapy followed by a stem cell transplant, when treated upon first presentation of the disease[7][8].

> *My dad was diagnosed with non-Hodgkin's lymphoma three years ago. It started with a knot in his lymph nodes in his neck. The doctor told him after treatment that it would probably not come back. His did, and it just keeps coming back in different places. Does non-Hodgkin's usually keep coming back in different places? Are the treatments just not getting it all and it moves? The doctors wanted him to do stem cell treatment; how good is that treatment and will it come back if you have that done?*

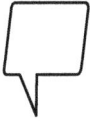

Non-Hodgkin's can come back in a different place to its initial site of presentation. Hodgkin's can as well, but is more likely to reoccur at the original site. Unfortunately, the treatments do not always get all the lymphoma cells, so it comes back. In some of the indolence lymphomas, where the periods of remission can be very long, there is a question of whether the whole process has simply started up again.

Immunotherapy

Immune-based therapy is dominated now by the oft used and effective rituximab monoclonal antibody, sold under the trade name Rituxan (or as Mabthera in Europe and Australia). Some say it is a landmark medicine. It can have good activity against mantle cell lymphoma alone but especially in combination with chemotherapies to prolong response duration. Rituximab essentially tags the cancer cells for destruction by the body. There are newer variations on monoclonal antibodies combined with radioactive molecules known as Radioimmunotherapy (RIT). These include Zevalin and Bexxar. Rituximab has also been used in small numbers of patients in combination with thalidomide with some effect.[9]

Targeted therapy

New targeted agents include the proteasome inhibitor Velcade and mTor inhibitors such as temsirolimus.

Epidemiology

Of all cancers involving the same class of blood cell, 6% of cases are mantle cell lymphoma.[10]

REFERENCES – LYMPHOMA

1. Parham, Peter (2005). *The immune system*. New York: Garland Science. p. 414. ISBN 0-8153-4093-1.

2. Hellman, Samuel; Mauch, P.M. Ed. (1999). *Hodgkin's Disease*. Chapter 1: Lippincott Williams & Wilkins. p. 5. ISBN 0-7817-1502-4.

3. Wagman LD. "Principles of Surgical Oncology" in Pazdur R, Wagman LD, Camphausen KA, Hoskins WJ (Eds) Cancer Management: A Multidisciplinary Approach. 11 ed. 2008.

4. ed. by Elaine S. Jaffe .... (2001). *Pathology and Genetics of Haemo (World Health Organization Classification of Tumours S.)*. Oxford Univ Pr. ISBN 92-832-2411-6.

5. www.emedicine.com on Lymphoma, Non-Hodgkin

6. http://www.crd.york.ac.uk/CRDWeb/ShowRecord.asp?ID=12005004101

REFERENCES – LYMPHOID LEUKEMIA

1. Parham, Peter (2005). *The immune system*. New York: Garland Science. p. 414. ISBN 0-8153-4093-1.

REFERENCES – HODGKIN'S LYMPHOMA

1. Hellman S. (2007). "Brief Consideration of Thomas Hodgkin and His Times". in Hoppe RT, Mauch PT, Armitage JO, Diehl V, Weiss LM. *Hodgkin's disease* (2nd ed.). Lippincott Williams & Wilkins. pp. 3–6. ISBN 978-0-7817-6422-3.

2. Fermé C, Eghbali H, Meerwaldt JH, et al. (November 2007). "Chemotherapy plus involved-field radiation in early-stage Hodgkin's disease". *The New England Journal of Medicine* **357** (19): 1916–27. doi:10.1056/NEJMoa064601. PMID 17989384. Lay summary – *HealthDay* (2007-11-07).

3. Stein, RS.; Morgan, D (2003). Handbook of Cancer Chemotherapy, Sixth Edition. Lippincott Williams & Wilkins, 493, Table 21.2: "Hodgkin's Disease: Incidence of stages and results of therapy." ISBN 0-7817-3629-3.

4. "HMDS: Hodgkin's Lymphoma". http://www.hmds.org.uk/hl.html. Retrieved on 2009-02-01.

5. Küppers R, Schwering I, Bräuninger A, Rajewsky K, Hansmann ML (2002). "Biology of Hodgkin's lymphoma". *Ann. Oncol.* **13** Suppl 1: 11–8. PMID 12078890. http://annonc.oxfordjournals.org/cgi/pmidlookup?view=long&pmid=12078890.

6. Bräuninger A, Schmitz R, Bechtel D, Renné C, Hansmann ML, Küppers R (April 2006). "Molecular biology of Hodgkin's and Reed/Sternberg cells in Hodgkin's lymphoma". *Int. J. Cancer* **118** (8): 1853–61. doi:10.1002/ijc.21716. PMID 16385563.

7. Tzankov A, Bourgau C, Kaiser A, *et al.* (December 2005). "Rare expression of T-cell markers in classical Hodgkin's lymphoma". *Mod. Pathol.* **18** (12): 1542–9. doi:10.1038/modpathol.3800473. PMID 16056244.

8. Lamprecht B, Kreher S, Anagnostopoulos, I, Johrens k, Monteleone G, Junt F, Stein H, Janz M, Dorken B, Mathas S (2008). "Aberrant expression of the Th2 cytokine IL-21 in Hodgkin lymphoma cells regulates STAT3 signaling and attracts Treg cells via regulation of MIP-3a". *Blood* **112** (Oct 2008): 3339–3347. doi:10.1182/blood-2008-01-134783. PMID 18684866. http://bloodjournal.hematologylibrary.org/cgi/content/abstract/112/8/3339.

9. Bobrove AM (June 1983). "Alcohol-related pain and Hodgkin's disease". *The Western Journal of Medicine* **138** (6): 874–5. PMID 6613116.

10. Portlock CS (July 2008). "Hodgkin Lymphoma". *Merck Manual Professional.* http://www.merck.com/mmpe/sec11/ch143/ch143b.html. Retrieved on 2009-06-18.

11. Hodgon DC, Gospodarowicz MK (2007). "Clinical Evaluation and Staging of Hodgkin Lymphoma". in Hoppe RT, Mauch PT, Armitage JO, Diehl V, Weiss LM. *Hodgkin's disease.* Lippincott Williams & Wilkins. pp. 123–132. ISBN 978-0-7817-6422-3.

12. Asher, Richard (July 6, 1995). "Making Sense". *The New England Journal of Medicine* **333**: 66–67. doi:10.1056/NEJM199507063330118. PMID 7777006.

13. Hodgkin's disease (Hodgkin's lymphoma) at Mount Sinai Hospital

14. Hasenclever D, Diehl V (1998-11-19). "A Prognostic Score for Advanced Hodgkin's Disease". *New England Journal of Medicine* **339** (21): 1506–14. doi:10.1056/NEJM199811193392104. PMID 9819449.

15. Gobbi PG, Levis A, Chisesi T, **et al.** (2005). "ABVD versus modified stanford V versus MOPPEBVCAD with optional and limited radiotherapy in intermediate- and advanced-stage Hodgkin's lymphoma: final results of a multicenter randomized trial by the Intergruppo Italiano Linfomi". *J. Clin. Oncol.* **23** (36): 9198–207. doi:10.1200/JCO.2005.02.907. PMID 16172458.

16. Home | German Hodgkin Study Group

17. Klimm B, Diehl V, Engert A (2007). "Hodgkin's Lymphoma in the Elderly: A Different Disease in Patients Over 60". *Oncology* **21** (8). http://www.cancernetwork.com/display/article/10165/59443.

18. Mauch, Peter; James Armitage, Volker Diehl, Richard Hoppe, Laurence Weiss (1999). *Hodgkin's Disease*. Lippincott Williams & Wilkins. pp. 62–64. ISBN 0-7817-1502-4.

19. Biggar RJ, Jaffe ES, Goedert JJ, Chaturvedi A, Pfeiffer R, Engels EA (2006). "Hodgkin lymphoma and immunodeficiency in persons with HIV/AIDS". *Blood* **108** (12): 3786–91. doi:10.1182/blood-2006-05-024109. PMID 16917006.

20. James, TGH (2004). "Carter, Howard (1874–1939)". *Oxford Dictionary of National Biography*. Oxford University Press. doi:10.1093/ref:odnb/32312.

21. "#41 Paul Allen". *The World's Billionaires*. Forbes. 2008-03-05. http://www.forbes.com/lists/2008/10/billionaires08_Paul-Allen_1217.html.

22. "Soul star dies after cancer fight". BBC News. http://news.bbc.co.uk/1/hi/entertainment/4716060.stm. Retrieved on 2008-12-27.

23. "Singer Goodrem has cancer". BBC News. http://news.bbc.co.uk/1/hi/entertainment/music/3057991.stm. Retrieved on 2008-12-27.

24. Ainley, Mark (2002). "Dinu Lipatti". http://www.markainley.com/music/classical/lipatti/prince_of_pianists.html.

25. Terry, MJ (2002). "Mario Lemieux". *Celebrity Survivor Biographies*. CureHodgkins. http://www.curehodgkins.com/hodgkins_resources/celebrity_survivors.html.

26. "Teen, court reach agreement over cancer care". Associated Press. MSNBC. 2006-09-05. http://www.msnbc.msn.com/id/14371567/. Retrieved on 2009-06-18.

27. "Big John Studd". *Hall of Fame*. WWE. http://www.wwe.com/superstars/halloffame/bigjohnstudd/bio/.

28. Shanahan M; Goldstein M (2009-05-19). "Time for 'Grown Ups'". Boston Globe. http://www.boston.com/ae/celebrity/articles/2009/05/19/time_for_grown_ ups/. Retrieved on 2009-06-18.

29. "Minnesota: Evaluation Ordered for a 13-Year-Old With Cancer". Associated Press. NY Times. 2009-05-16. http://www.nytimes.com/2009/05/16/us/16brfs-EVALUATIONOR_BRF.html?_r=1&scp=4&sq=daniel%20hauser&st=cse. Retrieved on 2009-06-18.

REFERENCES – NON-HODGKIN'S LYMPHOMA

1. *non-Hodgkin lymphomas* at Dorland's Medical Dictionary

2. ed. by Elaine S. Jaffe .... (2001). *Pathology and Genetics of Haemo (World Health Organization Classification of Tumours S.).* Oxford Univ Pr. ISBN 92-832-2411-6.

REFERENCES – BURKITT LYMPHOMA

1. synd/2511 at Who Named It?

2. Burkitt D (1958). "A sarcoma involving the jaws in African children". *The British journal of surgery* **46** (197): 218–23. doi:10.1002/bjs.18004619704. PMID 13628987.

3. Liu D, Shimonov J, Primanneni S, Lai Y, Ahmed T, Seiter K (2007). "t(8;14;18): a 3-way chromosome translocation in two patients with Burkitt's lymphoma/leukemia". *Mol. Cancer* **6**: 35. doi:10.1186/1476-4598-6-35. PMID 17547754.

4. Smardova J, Grochova D, Fabian P, et al. (October 2008). "An unusual p53 mutation detected in Burkitt's lymphoma: 30 bp duplication". *Oncol. Rep.* **20** (4): 773–8. PMID 18813817. http://www.spandidos-publications.com/or/article.jsp?article_id=or_20_4_773.

5. Ferry JA (April 2006). "Burkitt's lymphoma: clinicopathologic features and differential diagnosis". *Oncologist* **11** (4): 375–83. doi:10.1634/theoncologist.11-4-375. PMID 16614233. http://theoncologist.alphamedpress.org/cgi/pmidlookup?view=long&pmid=16614233.

6. Bellan C, Lazzi S, De Falco G, Nyongo A, Giordano A, Leoncini L (March 2003). "Burkitt's lymphoma: new insights into molecular pathogenesis". *J. Clin. Pathol.* **56** (3): 188–92. doi:10.1136/jcp.56.3.188. PMID 12610094. PMC: 1769902. http://jcp.bmj.com/cgi/pmidlookup?view=long&pmid=12610094.

7. Fujita S, Buziba N, Kumatori A, Senba M, Yamaguchi A, Toriyama K (May 2004). "Early stage of Epstein-Barr virus lytic infection leading to the "starry sky" pattern formation in endemic Burkitt lymphoma". *Arch. Pathol. Lab. Med.* **128** (5): 549–52. PMID 15086279. http://journals.allenpress.com/jrnlserv/?request=get-abstract&issn=0003-9985&volume=128&page=549.

8. Wyndham H. Wilson, Kieron Dunleavy, Stefania Pittaluga, Upendra Hegde, Nicole Grant, Seth M. Steinberg, Mark Raffeld, Martin Gutierrez, Bruce A. Chabner, Louis Staudt, Elaine S. Jaffe, and John E. Janik (2008). "Phase II Study of Dose-Adjusted EPOCH-Rituximab in Untreated Diffuse Large B-cell Lymphoma with Analysis of Germinal Center and Post-Germinal Center Biomarkers". *Journal of Clinical Oncology* **26** (16): 2717–2714. doi:10.1200/JCO.2007.13.1391. PMID 18378569.

9. Yustein JT, Dang CV (2007). "Biology and treatment of Burkitt's lymphoma". *Curr. Opin. Hematol.* **14** (4): 375–81. doi:10.1097/MOH.0b013e3281bccdee. PMID 17534164.

10. Turgeon, Mary Louise (2005). *Clinical hematology: theory and procedures.* Hagerstown, MD: Lippincott Williams & Wilkins. pp. 283. ISBN 0-7817-5007-5. "Frequency of lymphoid neoplasms. (Source: Modified from WHO Blue Book on Tumour of Hematopoietic and Lymphoid Tissues. 2001, p. 2001.)"

REFERENCES – WALDLENSTROM'S MACROGLOBULINEMIA

1. Cheson BD (2006). "Chronic Lymphoid Leukemias and Plasma Cell Disorders". in Dale DD, Federman DD. *ACP Medicine*. New York, NY: WebMD Professional Publishing. ISBN 0974832715.

2. Waldenstrom J (1944). "Incipient myelomatosis or "essential" hyperglobulinemia with fibrinognenopenia-a new syndrome?". *Acta Med Scand* **117**: 216–247.

3. Harris NL, Jaffe ES, Diebold J, Flandrin G, Muller-Hermelink HK, Vardiman J, Lister TA, Bloomfield CD (2000). "The World Health Organization classification of neoplastic diseases of the haematopoietic and lymphoid tissues: Report of the Clinical Advisory Committee Meeting, Airlie House, Virginia, November 1997". *Histopathology* **36** (1): 69–86. doi:10.1046/j.1365-2559.2000.00895.x. PMID 10632755.

4. Schop RF, Van Wier SA, Xu R, et al. (2006). "6q deletion discriminates Waldenström macroglobulinemia from IgM monoclonal gammopathy of undetermined significance". *Cancer Genet. Cytogenet.* **169** (2): 150–3. doi:10.1016/j.cancergencyto.2006.04.009. PMID 16938573.

5. PMID 18809818

6. PMID 18703425

7. http://www.asco.org/ASCO/Abstracts+&+Virtual+Meeting/Abstracts?&vmview=abst_detail_view&confID=26&abstractID=4297

8. doi:10.1182/blood-2007-05-092098

9. PMID 14612935

10. PMID 18334673

11. doi:10.1038/sj.leu.2404520

12. PMID 18516762

13. PMID 16804116

14. PMID 12720156

15. Turgeon, Mary Louise (2005). *Clinical hematology: theory and procedures*. Hagerstown, MD: Lippincott Williams & Wilkins. p. 283. ISBN 0-7817-5007-5. "Frequency of lymphoid neoplasms. (Source: Modified from WHO Blue Book on Tumour of Hematopoietic and Lymphoid Tissues. 2001, p. 2001.)"

16. Raje N, Hideshima T, Anderson KC (2003). "Plasma Cell Tumors". in Kufe DW, Pollock RE, Weichselbaum RR, Bast RC, Gansler TS. *Holland-Frei Cancer Medicine* (6th ed.). New York, NY: B.C. Decker. ISBN 1550092138.

17. Kyle RA (1998). "Chapter 94: Multiple Myeloma and the Dysproteinemias". in Stein JH. *Internal Medicine* (5th ed.). New York: C.V.Mosby. ISBN 0815186983.

18. Owen RG, Barrans SL, Richards SJ, O'Connor SJ, Child JA, Parapia LA, Morgan GJ, Jack AS (2001). "Waldenstrom macroglobulinemia. Development of diagnostic criteria and identification of prognostic factors". *Am J Clin Pathol* **116** (3): 420–8. doi:10.1309/4LCN-JMPG-5U71-UWQB. PMID 11554171.

19. San Miguel JF, Vidriales MB, Ocio E, Mateo G, Sanchez-Guijo F, Sanchez ML, Escribano L, Barez A, Moro MJ, Hernandez J, Aguilera C, Cuello R, Garcia-Frade J, Lopez R, Portero J, Orfao A (2003). "Immunophenotypic analysis of Waldenstrom's macroglobulinemia". *Semin Oncol* **30** (2): 187–95. doi:10.1053/sonc.2003.50074. PMID 12720134.

20. Ghobrial IM, Witzig TE (2004). "Waldenstrom macroglobulinemia". *Curr Treat Options Oncol* **5** (3): 239–47. doi:10.1007/s11864-004-0015-5. PMID 15115652.

21. Dimopoulos MA, Kyle RA, Anagnostopoulos A, Treon SP (2005). "Diagnosis and management of Waldenstrom's macroglobulinemia". *J Clin Oncol* **23** (7): 1564–77. doi:10.1200/JCO.2005.03.144. PMID 15735132.

22. http://emedicine.medscape.com/article/207097-overview

23. Johansson B, Waldenstrom J, Hasselblom S, Mitelman F (1995). "Waldenstrom's macroglobulinemia with the AML/MDS-associated t(1;3)(p36;q21)". *Leukemia* **9** (7): 1136–8. PMID 7630185.

24. Morel P, Duhamel A, Gobbi P, Dimopoulos M, Dhodapkar M, McCoy J, *et al*. International Prognostic Scoring System for Waldenström's Macroglobulinemia. XIth International Myeloma Workshop & IVth International Workshop on Waldenstrom's Macroglobulinemia 25 30 June 2007 Kos Island, Greece. Haematologica 2007;92(6 suppl 2):1-229.

25. PMID 18641029

26. PMID 18931340

27. PMID 19087134

28. Waldenstrom J (1991). "To treat or not to treat, this is the real question". *Leuk Res* **15** (6): 407–8. doi:10.1016/0145-2126(91)90049-Y. PMID 1907339.

29. http://emedicine.medscape.com/article/207097-treatment

30. PMID 18813229

31. Kyle RA, Treon SP, Alexanian R, Barlogie B, Bjorkholm M, Dhodapkar M, Lister TA, Merlini G, Morel P, Stone M, Branagan AR, Leblond V (2003). "Prognostic markers and criteria to initiate therapy in Waldenstrom's macroglobulinemia: consensus panel recommendations from the Second International Workshop on Waldenstrom's Macroglobulinemia". *Semin Oncol* **30** (2): 116–20. doi:10.1053/sonc.2003.50038. PMID 12720119.

32. PMID 18713945

33. Gertz MA (2005). "Waldenstrom macroglobulinemia: a review of therapy". *Am J Hematol* **79** (2): 147–57. doi:10.1002/ajh.20363. PMID 15929102.

34. Yang L, Wen B, Li H, Yang M, Jin Y, Yang S, Tao J (1999). "Autologous peripheral blood stem cell transplantation for Waldenstrom's macroglobulinemia". *Bone Marrow Transplant* **24** (8): 929–30. doi:10.1038/sj.bmt.1701992. PMID 10516708.

35. Martino R, Shah A, Romero P, Brunet S, Sierra J, Domingo-Albos A, Fruchtman S, Isola L (1999). "Allogeneic bone marrow transplantation for advanced Waldenstrom's macroglobulinemia". *Bone Marrow Transplant* **23** (7): 747–9. doi:10.1038/sj.bmt.1701633. PMID 10218857.

36. Anagnostopoulos A, Dimopoulos MA, Aleman A, Weber D, Alexanian R, Champlin R, Giralt S (2001). "High-dose chemotherapy followed by stem cell transplantation in patients with resistant Waldenstrom's macroglobulinemia". *Bone Marrow Transplant* **27** (10): 1027–9. doi:10.1038/sj.bmt.1703041. PMID 11438816.

37. Tournilhac O, Leblond V, Tabrizi R, Gressin R, Senecal D, Milpied N, Cazin B, Divine M, Dreyfus B, Cahn JY, Pignon B, Desablens B, Perrier JF, Bay JO, Travade P (2003). "Transplantation in Waldenstrom's macroglobulinemia--the French experience". *Semin Oncol* **30** (2): 291–6. doi:10.1053/sonc.2003.50048. PMID 12720155.

38. http://clinicaltrials.gov/ct2/results?term=Waldenstrom

39. ClinicalTrials.gov NCT00608374

40. ClinicalTrials.gov NCT00566332

41. [1]

REFERENCES – PRIMARY EFFUSION LYMPHOMA

1. *primary effusion lymphoma* at Dorland's Medical Dictionary

2. Cesarman E, Chang Y, Moore PS, Said JW, Knowles DM (May 1995). "Kaposi's sarcoma-associated herpesvirus-like DNA sequences in AIDS-related body-cavity-based lymphomas". *N. Engl. J. Med.* **332** (18): 1186–91. doi:10.1056/NEJM199505043321802. PMID 7700311. http://content.nejm.org/cgi/pmidlook up?view=short&pmid=7700311&promo=ONFLNS19.

3. Staudt MR, Kanan Y, Jeong JH, Papin JF, Hines-Boykin R, Dittmer DP (July 2004). "The tumor microenvironment controls primary effusion lymphoma growth in vivo". *Cancer Res.* **64** (14): 4790–9. doi:10.1158/0008-5472.CAN-03-3835. PMID 15256448. http://cancerres.aacrjournals.org/cgi/pmidlookup?view =long&pmid=15256448.

4. Fan W, Bubman D, Chadburn A, Harrington WJ, Cesarman E, Knowles DM (January 2005). "Distinct subsets of primary effusion lymphoma can be identified based on their cellular gene expression profile and viral association". *J. Virol.* **79** (2): 1244–51. doi:10.1128/JVI.79.2.1244-1251.2005. PMID 15613351. PMC: 538532. http://jvi.asm.org/cgi/pmidlookup?view=long&pmid= 15613351.

5. Boshoff C, Weiss R (May 2002). "AIDS-related malignancies". *Nat. Rev. Cancer* **2** (5): 373–82. doi:10.1038/nrc797. PMID 12044013.

6. Yarchoan R, Tosato G, Little RF (August 2005). "Therapy insight: AIDS-related malignancies--the influence of antiviral therapy on pathogenesis and management". *Nat Clin Pract Oncol* **2** (8): 406–15; quiz 423. doi:10.1038/ncponc0253. PMID 16130937.

7. Youngster I, Vaisben E, Cohen H, Nassar F (January 2006). "An unusual cause of pleural effusion". *Age Ageing* **35** (1): 94–6. doi:10.1093/ageing/afj009. PMID 16364944. http://ageing.oxfordjournals.org/cgi/pmidlookup?view=long&pmid =16364944.

8. "Case 98-3 - AIDS-Related Primary Effusion Lymphoma". http://www.healthsystem.virginia.edu/internet/pathology/casestudies/heme/k98_3.cfm.

9. Chen YB, Rahemtullah A, Hochberg E (May 2007). "Primary effusion lymphoma". *Oncologist* **12** (5): 569–76. doi:10.1634/theoncologist.12-5-569. PMID 17522245. http://theoncologist.alphamedpress.org/cgi/pmidlookup?vie w=long&pmid=17522245.

10. Sin SH, Roy D, Wang L, *et al.* (March 2007). "Rapamycin is efficacious against primary effusion lymphoma (PEL) cell lines in vivo by inhibiting autocrine signaling". *Blood* **109** (5): 2165–73. doi:10.1182/blood-2006-06-028092. PMID 17082322. PMC: 1801055. http://www.bloodjournal.org/cgi/pmidlookup?view= long&pmid=17082322.

REFERENCES – SPLENIC MARGINAL ZONE LYMPHOMA

1. Elaine Sarkin Jaffe, Nancy Lee Harris, World Health Organization, International Agency for Research on Cancer, Harald Stein, J.W. Vardiman (2001). *Pathology and genetics of tumours of haematopoietic and lymphoid tissues.* World Health Organization Classification of Tumors. **3**. Lyon: IARC Press. ISBN 92-832-2411-6. http://books.google.com.au/books?id=XSKqcy7TUZUC.

2. Melo JV, Hegde U, Parreira A, Thompson I, Lampert IA, Catovsky D (June 1987). "Splenic B cell lymphoma with circulating villous lymphocytes: differential diagnosis of B cell leukaemias with large spleens". *J. Clin. Pathol.* **40** (6): 642–51. doi:10.1136/jcp.40.6.642. PMID 3497180. PMC: 1141055. http://jcp.bmj.com/cgi/pmidlookup?view=long&pmid=3497180.

3. Berger F, Felman P, Thieblemont C, *et al.* (March 2000). "Non-MALT marginal zone B-cell lymphomas: a description of clinical presentation and outcome in 124 patients". *Blood* **95** (6): 1950–6. PMID 10706860. http://www.bloodjournal.org/cgi/pmidlookup?view=long&pmid=10706860.

4. Mollejo M, Menárguez J, Lloret E, *et al.* (October 1995). "Splenic marginal zone lymphoma: a distinctive type of low-grade B-cell lymphoma. A clinicopathological study of 13 cases". *Am. J. Surg. Pathol.* **19** (10): 1146–57. PMID 7573673.

5. Jaffe ES, Costa J, Fauci AS, Cossman J, Tsokos M (November 1983). "Malignant lymphoma and erythrophagocytosis simulating malignant histiocytosis". *Am. J. Med.* **75** (5): 741–9. doi:10.1016/0002-9343(83)90402-3. PMID 6638043.

6. Franco V, Florena AM, Campesi G (December 1996). "Intrasinusoidal bone marrow infiltration: a possible hallmark of splenic lymphoma". *Histopathology* **29** (6): 571–5. doi:10.1046/j.1365-2559.1996.d01-536.x. PMID 8971565.

7. Isaacson PG, Matutes E, Burke M, Catovsky D (01 December 1994). "The histopathology of splenic lymphoma with villous lymphocytes". *Blood* **84** (11): 3828–34. PMID 7949139. http://www.bloodjournal.org/cgi/pmidlookup?view=long&pmid=7949139.

8. Matutes E, Morilla R, Owusu-Ankomah K, Houlihan A, Catovsky D (15 March 1994). "The immunophenotype of splenic lymphoma with villous lymphocytes and its relevance to the differential diagnosis with other B-cell disorders". *Blood* **83** (6): 1558–62. PMID 8123845. http://www.bloodjournal.org/cgi/pmidlookup?view=long&pmid=8123845.

9. Savilo E, Campo E, Mollejo M, *et al.* (July 1998). "Absence of cyclin D1 protein expression in splenic marginal zone lymphoma". *Mod. Pathol.* **11** (7): 601–6. PMID 9688179.

10. Dunn-Walters DK, Boursier L, Spencer J, Isaacson PG (June 1998). "Analysis of immunoglobulin genes in splenic marginal zone lymphoma suggests ongoing mutation". *Hum. Pathol.* **29** (6): 585–93. doi:10.1016/S0046-8177(98)80007-5. PMID 9635678.

11. Corcoran MM, Mould SJ, Orchard JA, et al. (November 1999). "Dysregulation of cyclin dependent kinase 6 expression in splenic marginal zone lymphoma through chromosome 7q translocations". *Oncogene* **18** (46): 6271–7. doi:10.1038/sj.onc.120303310.1038/sj.onc.1203033 (inactive 2009-06-29). PMID 10597225.

12. Armitage JO, Weisenburger DD (August 1998). "New approach to classifying non-Hodgkin's lymphomas: clinical features of the major histologic subtypes. Non-Hodgkin's Lymphoma Classification Project". *J. Clin. Oncol.* **16** (8): 2780–95. PMID 9704731. http://www.jco.org/cgi/pmidlookup?view=long&pmid=9704731.

REFERENCES – GASTRIC LYMPHOMA

1. Dawson IMP, Cornes JS, Morrison BC. Primary malignant lymphoid tumours of the intestinal tract. *Br J Surg*. 1961;49:80-89.

2. Aisenberg AC. Coherent view of non-Hodgkin's lymphoma. *J Clin Oncol*. 1995;13:2656-2675.

3. Koch P et al. Primary gastrointestinal non-Hodgkin's lymphoma: I. Anatomic and histologic distribution, clinical features, and survival data of 371 patients registered in the German Multicenter Study GIT NHL 01/92. *J Clin Oncol* 2001 Sep 15;19(18):3861-73.

4. Thirlby RC. Gastrointestinal lymphoma: a surgical perspective. Oncology (Huntingt). 1993;7:29-32.

5. NEJM article

6. Bayerdorffer E et al., Regression of primary gastric lymphoma of mucosa-associated lymphoid tissue type after cure of Helicobacter pylori infection. MALT Lymphoma Study Group, *Lancet* 1995 Jun 24;345(8965):1591-4.

7. Hammel P et al. Efficacy of single-agent chemotherapy in low-grade B-cell mucosa-associated lymphoid tissue lymphoma with prominent gastric expression. *J Clin Oncol* 1995 Oct;13(10):2524-9.

REFERENCES – FOLLICULAR LYMPHOMA

1. Overview at UMDNJ

2. Barekman CL, Aguilera NS, Abbondanzo SL (July 2001). "Low-grade B-cell lymphoma with coexpression of both CD5 and CD10. A report of 3 cases". *Arch. Pathol. Lab. Med.* **125** (7): 951–3. PMID 11419985. http://journals. allenpress.com/jrnlserv/?request=get-abstract&issn=0003-9985&volume=125 &page=951.

3. *follicular lymphoma* at Dorland's Medical Dictionary

4. "Follicular Lymphomas". http://pleiad.umdnj.edu/hemepath/follicular/ follicular.html. Retrieved on 2008-07-26.

5. Bosga-Bouwer AG, van Imhoff GW, Boonstra R, *et al.* (February 2003). "Follicular lymphoma grade 3B includes 3 cytogenetically defined subgroups with primary t(14;18), 3q27, or other translocations: t(14;18) and 3q27 are mutually exclusive". *Blood* **101** (3): 1149–54. doi:10.1182/blood.V101.3.1149. PMID 12529293. http://www.bloodjournal.org/cgi/pmidlookup?view=long&p mid=12529293.

6. Bosga-Bouwer AG, Haralambieva E, Booman M, et al. (November 2005). "BCL6 alternative translocation breakpoint cluster region associated with follicular lymphoma grade 3B". *Genes Chromosomes Cancer* **44** (3): 301–4. doi:10.1002/ gcc.20246. PMID 16075463.

7. Turgeon, Mary Louise (2005). *Clinical hematology: theory and procedures.* Hagerstown, MD: Lippincott Williams & Wilkins. p. 283. ISBN 0-7817-5007-5. "Frequency of lymphoid neoplasms. (Source: Modified from WHO Blue Book on Tumour of Hematopoietic and Lymphoid Tissues. 2001, p. 2001.)"

REFERENCES – ANAPLASTIC LARGE CELL LYMPHOMA

1. Balamurugan S, Rajasekar B, Rao RR (2009). "Anaplastic large-cell lymphoma with florid granulomatous reaction: A case report and review of literature". *Indian J Pathol Microbiol* **52** (1): 69–70. PMID 19136786. http://www.ijpmonline. org/article.asp?issn=0377-4929;year=2009;volume=52;issue=1;spage=69;epag e=70;aulast=Balamurugan.

2. Watanabe M, Ogawa Y, Itoh K, *et al.* (January 2008). "Hypomethylation of CD30 CpG islands with aberrant JunB expression drives CD30 induction in Hodgkin lymphoma and anaplastic large cell lymphoma". *Lab. Invest.* **88** (1): 48–57. doi:10.1038/labinvest.3700696. PMID 17965727. http://dx.doi.org/10.1038/ labinvest.3700696.

3. Park SJ, Kim S, Lee DH, *et al.* (August 2008). "Primary systemic anaplastic large cell lymphoma in Korean adults: 11 years' experience at Asan Medical Center". *Yonsei Med. J.* **49** (4): 601–9. doi:10.3349/ymj.2008.49.4.601. PMID 18729302. http://www.eymj.org/abstracts/viewArticle. asp?year=2008&page=601.

4. de Jong D, Vasmel WL, de Boer JP, *et al.* (November 2008). "Anaplastic large-cell lymphoma in women with breast implants". *JAMA* **300** (17): 2030–5. doi:10.1001/jama.2008.585. PMID 18984890.

REFERENCES – PRIMARY CNS LYMPHOMA

1. Fine HA, Mayer RJ. Primary central nervous system lymphoma. *Ann Intern Med* 1993; 119(11):1093-1104

2. Eby NL, Grufferman S, Flannelly CM, Schold SC, Jr., Vogel FS, Burger PC. Increasing incidence of primary brain lymphoma in the US. *Cancer* 1988;62(11):2461-2465

3. Corn BW, Marcus SM, Topham A, Hauck W, Curran WJ, Jr. Will primary central nervous system lymphoma be the most frequent brain tumor diagnosed in the year 2000? *Cancer* 1997;79(12):2409-2413

4. Lukes RJ, Collins RD. Immunologic characterization of human malignant lymphomas. *Cancer* 1974;34:1488-1503

5. Jellinger K, Radaskiewictz T, Slowik F. Primary malignant lymphomas of the central nervous system in man. *Acta Neuropathol* 1975;95-102 (suppl 6)

6. Herrlinger U, Schabet M, Bitzer M, Petersen D, Krauseneck P. Primary central nervous system lymphoma: from clinical presentation to diagnosis. *J Neurosurg* 2000; 92:261-266

7. Herrlinger U, Schabet M, Bitzer M, Petersen D, Krauseneck P. Primary central nervous system lymphoma: from clinical presentation to diagnosis. *J.Neurooncol.* 1999;43:219-226. (PMID: 10563426).

8. Deangelis LM, Hormigo A. Treatment of primary central nervous system lymphoma. *Semin Oncol* 2004; 31:684-692.

REFERENCES – MANTLE CELL LYMPHOMA

1. Mantle Cell Lymphoma

2. t(11;14)(q13;q32)

3. Li JY, Gaillard F, Moreau A, *et al.* (May 1999). "Detection of translocation t(11;14)(q13;q32) in mantle cell lymphoma by fluorescence in situ hybridization". *Am. J. Pathol.* **154** (5): 1449–52. PMID 10329598. PMC: 1866594. http://ajp.amjpathol.org/cgi/pmidlookup?view=long&pmid=10329598.

4. Barouk-Simonet E, Andrieux J, Copin MC, *et al.* (2002). "TPA stimulation culture for improved detection of t(11;14)(q13;q32) in mantle cell lymphoma". *Ann. Genet.* **45** (3): 165–8. PMID 12381451. http://linkinghub.elsevier.com/retrieve/pii/S000339950201122X.

5. Mantle Cell Lymphoma: An Update for Clinicians [1]

6. Stanford School of Medicine: "Mantle Cell Lymphoma, Differential Diagnosis" [2]

7. Barekman CL, Aguilera NS, Abbondanzo SL (July 2001). "Low-grade B-cell lymphoma with coexpression of both CD5 and CD10. A report of 3 cases". *Arch. Pathol. Lab. Med.* **125** (7): 951–3. PMID 11419985. http://journals. allenpress.com/jrnlserv/?request=get-abstract&issn=0003-9985&volume=125 &page=951.

8. Hoster *et al.* A new prognostic index (MIPI) for patients with advanced-stage mantle cell lymphoma. Blood 2008;111:558-565.

9. Kaufmann, Hannes; Markus Raderer, Stefan Wöhrer, Andreas Püspök, Alexander Bankier, Christoph Zielinski, Andreas Chott, Johannes Drach (15 October 2004). "Antitumor activity of rituximab plus thalidomide in patients with relapsed/refractory mantle cell lymphoma" (PDF). *Blood* **104** (8): 2269–71. doi:10.1182/blood-2004-03-1091. http://bloodjournal.hematologylibrary.org/cgi/reprint/104/8/2269. Retrieved on 2008-02-13.

10. Turgeon, Mary Louise (2005). *Clinical hematology: theory and procedures.* Hagerstown, MD: Lippincott Williams & Wilkins. pp. 283. ISBN 0-7817-5007-5. "Frequency of lymphoid neoplasms. (Source: Modified from WHO Blue Book on Tumour of Hematopoietic and Lymphoid Tissues. 2001, p. 2001.)"

GNU FREE DOCUMENTATION LICENSE

0. PREAMBLE

The purpose of this License is to make a manual, textbook, or other functional and useful document "free" in the sense of freedom: to assure everyone the effective freedom to copy and redistribute it, with or without modifying it, either commercially or noncommercially. Secondarily, this License preserves for the author and publisher a way to get credit for their work, while not being considered responsible for modifications made by others.

This License is a kind of "copyleft", which means that derivative works of the document must themselves be free in the same sense. It complements the GNU General Public License, which is a copyleft license designed for free software.

We have designed this License in order to use it for manuals for free software, because free software needs free documentation: a free program should come with manuals providing the same freedoms that the software does. But this License is not limited to software manuals; it can be used for any textual work, regardless of subject matter or whether it is published as a printed book. We recommend this License principally for works whose purpose is instruction or reference.

1. APPLICABILITY AND DEFINITIONS

This License applies to any manual or other work, in any medium, that contains a notice placed by the copyright holder saying it can be distributed under the terms of this License. Such a notice grants a world-wide, royalty-free license, unlimited in duration, to use that work under the conditions stated herein. The "Document", herein, refers to any such manual or work. Any member of the public is a licensee, and is addressed as "you". You accept the license if you copy, modify or distribute the work in a way requiring permission under copyright law.

A "Modified Version" of the Document means any work containing the Document or a portion of it, either copied verbatim, or with modifications and/or translated into another language.

A "Secondary Section" is a named appendix or a front-matter section of the Document that deals exclusively with the relationship of the publishers or authors of the Document to the Document's overall subject (or to related matters) and contains nothing that could fall directly within that overall subject. (Thus, if the Document is in part a textbook of mathematics, a Secondary Section may not explain any mathematics.) The relationship could be a matter of historical connection with the subject or with related matters, or of legal, commercial, philosophical, ethical or political position regarding them.

The "Invariant Sections" are certain Secondary Sections whose titles are designated, as being those of Invariant Sections, in the notice that says that the Document is released under this License. If a section does not fit the above definition of Secondary then it is not allowed to be designated as Invariant. The Document may contain zero Invariant Sections. If the Document does not identify any Invariant Sections then there are none.

The "Cover Texts" are certain short passages of text that are listed, as Front-Cover Texts or Back-Cover Texts, in the notice that says that the Document is released under this License. A Front-Cover Text may be at most 5 words, and a Back-Cover Text may be at most 25 words.

A "Transparent" copy of the Document means a machine-readable copy, represented in a format whose specification is available to the general public, that is suitable for revising the document straightforwardly with generic text editors or (for images composed of pixels) generic paint programs or (for drawings) some widely available drawing editor, and that is suitable for input to text formatters or for automatic translation to a variety of formats suitable for input to text formatters. A copy made in an otherwise Transparent file format whose markup, or absence of markup, has been arranged to thwart or discourage subsequent modification by readers is not Transparent. An image format is not Transparent if used for any substantial amount of text. A copy that is not "Transparent" is called "Opaque".

Examples of suitable formats for Transparent copies include plain ASCII without markup, Texinfo input format, LaTeX input format, SGML or XML using a publicly available DTD, and standard-conforming simple HTML, PostScript or PDF designed for human modification. Examples of transparent image formats include PNG, XCF and JPG. Opaque formats include proprietary formats that can be read and edited only by proprietary word processors, SGML or XML for which the DTD and/or processing tools are not generally available, and the machine-generated HTML, PostScript or PDF produced by some word processors for output purposes only.

The "Title Page" means, for a printed book, the title page itself, plus such following pages as are needed to hold, legibly, the material this License requires to appear in the title page. For works in formats which do not have any title page as such, "Title Page" means the text near the most prominent appearance of the work's title, preceding the beginning of the body of the text.

A section "Entitled XYZ" means a named subunit of the Document whose title either is precisely XYZ or contains XYZ in parentheses following text that translates XYZ in another language. (Here XYZ stands for a specific section name mentioned below, such as "Acknowledgements", "Dedications", "Endorsements", or "History".) To "Preserve the Title" of such a section when you modify the Document means that it remains a section "Entitled XYZ" according to this definition.

The Document may include Warranty Disclaimers next to the notice which states that this License applies to the Document. These Warranty Disclaimers are considered to be included by reference in this License, but only as regards disclaiming warranties: any other implication that these Warranty Disclaimers may have is void and has no effect on the meaning of this License.

2. VERBATIM COPYING

You may copy and distribute the Document in any medium, either commercially or noncommercially, provided that this License, the copyright notices, and the license notice saying this License applies to the Document are reproduced in all copies, and that you add no other conditions whatsoever to those of this License. You may not use technical measures to obstruct or control the reading or further copying of the copies you make or distribute. However, you may accept compensation in exchange for copies. If you distribute a large enough number of copies you must also follow the conditions in section 3.

You may also lend copies, under the same conditions stated above, and you may publicly display copies.

3. COPYING IN QUANTITY

If you publish printed copies (or copies in media that commonly have printed covers) of the Document, numbering more than 100, and the Document's license notice requires Cover Texts, you must enclose the copies in covers that carry, clearly and legibly, all these Cover Texts: Front-Cover Texts on the front cover, and Back-Cover Texts on the back cover. Both covers must also clearly and legibly identify you as the publisher of these copies. The front cover must present the full title with all words of the title equally prominent and visible. You may add other material on the covers in addition. Copying with changes limited to the covers, as long as they preserve the title of the Document and satisfy these conditions, can be treated as verbatim copying in other respects.

If the required texts for either cover are too voluminous to fit legibly, you should put the first ones listed (as many as fit reasonably) on the actual cover, and continue the rest onto adjacent pages.

If you publish or distribute Opaque copies of the Document numbering more than 100, you must either include a machine-readable Transparent copy along with each Opaque copy, or state in or with each Opaque copy a computer-network location from which the general network-using public has access to download using public-standard network protocols a complete Transparent copy of the Document, free of added material. If you use the latter option, you must take reasonably prudent steps, when you begin distribution of Opaque copies in quantity, to ensure that this Transparent copy will remain thus accessible at the stated location until at least one year after the last time you distribute an Opaque copy (directly or through your agents or retailers) of that edition to the public.

It is requested, but not required, that you contact the authors of the Document well before redistributing any large number of copies, to give them a chance to provide you with an updated version of the Document.

4. MODIFICATIONS

You may copy and distribute a Modified Version of the Document under the conditions of sections 2 and 3 above, provided that you release the Modified Version under precisely this License, with the Modified Version filling the role of the Document, thus licensing distribution and modification of the Modified Version to whoever possesses a copy of it. In addition, you must do these things in the Modified Version:

A. Use in the Title Page (and on the covers, if any) a title distinct from that of the Document, and from those of previous versions (which should, if there were any, be listed in the History section of the Document). You may use the same title as a previous version if the original publisher of that version gives permission.

B. List on the Title Page, as authors, one or more persons or entities responsible for authorship of the modifications in the Modified Version, together with at least five of the principal authors of the Document (all of its principal authors, if it has fewer than five), unless they release you from this requirement.

C. State on the Title page the name of the publisher of the Modified Version, as the publisher.

D. Preserve all the copyright notices of the Document.

E. Add an appropriate copyright notice for your modifications adjacent to the other copyright notices.

F. Include, immediately after the copyright notices, a license notice giving the public permission to use the Modified Version under the terms of this License, in the form shown in the Addendum below.

G. Preserve in that license notice the full lists of Invariant Sections and required Cover Texts given in the Document's license notice.

H. Include an unaltered copy of this License.

I. Preserve the section Entitled "History", Preserve its Title, and add to it an item stating at least the title, year, new authors, and publisher of the Modified Version as given on the Title Page. If there is no section Entitled "History" in the Document, create one stating the title, year, authors, and publisher of the Document as given on its Title Page, then add an item describing the Modified Version as stated in the previous sentence.

J. Preserve the network location, if any, given in the Document for public access to a Transparent copy of the Document, and likewise the network locations given in the Document for previous versions it was based on. These may be placed in the "History" section. You may omit a network location for a work that was published at least four years before the Document itself, or if the original publisher of the version it refers to gives permission.

K. For any section entitled "Acknowledgements" or "Dedications", Preserve the Title of the section, and preserve in the section all the substance and tone of each of the contributor acknowledgements and/or dedications given therein.

L. Preserve all the Invariant Sections of the Document, unaltered in their text and in their titles. Section numbers or the equivalent are not considered part of the section titles.

M. Delete any section entitled "Endorsements". Such a section may not be included in the Modified Version.

N. Do not retitle any existing section to be entitled "Endorsements" or to conflict in title with any Invariant Section.

O. Preserve any Warranty Disclaimers.

If the Modified Version includes new front-matter sections or appendices that qualify as Secondary Sections and contain no material copied from the Document, you may at your option designate some or all of these sections as Invariant. To do this, add their titles to the list of Invariant Sections in the Modified Version's license notice. These titles must be distinct from any other section titles.

You may add a section entitled "Endorsements", provided it contains nothing but endorsements of your Modified Version by various parties—for example, statements of peer review or that the text has been approved by an organization as the authoritative definition of a standard.

You may add a passage of up to five words as a Front-Cover Text, and a passage of up to 25 words as a Back-Cover Text, to the end of the list of Cover Texts in the Modified Version. Only one passage of Front-Cover Text and one of Back-Cover Text may be added by (or through arrangements made by) any one entity. If the Document already includes a Cover Text for the same cover, previously added by you or by arrangement made by the same entity you are acting on behalf of, you may not add another; but you may replace the old one, on explicit permission from the previous publisher that added the old one.

The author(s) and publisher(s) of the Document do not by this License give permission to use their names for publicity for or to assert or imply endorsement of any Modified Version.

5. COMBINING DOCUMENTS

You may combine the Document with other documents released under this License, under the terms defined in section 4 above for modified versions, provided that you include in the combination all of the Invariant Sections of all of the original documents, unmodified, and list them all as Invariant Sections of your combined work in its license notice, and that you preserve all their Warranty Disclaimers.

The combined work need only contain one copy of this License, and multiple identical Invariant Sections may be replaced with a single copy. If there are multiple Invariant Sections with the same name but different contents, make the title of each such section unique by adding at the end of it, in parentheses, the name of the original author or publisher of that section if known, or else a unique number. Make the same adjustment to the section titles in the list of Invariant Sections in the license notice of the combined work.

In the combination, you must combine any sections entitled "History" in the various original documents, forming one section entitled "History";

likewise combine any sections entitled "Acknowledgements", and any sections entitled "Dedications". You must delete all sections entitled "Endorsements."

6. COLLECTIONS OF DOCUMENTS

You may make a collection consisting of the Document and other documents released under this License, and replace the individual copies of this License in the various documents with a single copy that is included in the collection, provided that you follow the rules of this License for verbatim copying of each of the documents in all other respects.

You may extract a single document from such a collection, and distribute it individually under this License, provided you insert a copy of this License into the extracted document, and follow this License in all other respects regarding verbatim copying of that document.

7. AGGREGATION WITH INDEPENDENT WORKS

A compilation of the Document or its derivatives with other separate and independent documents or works, in or on a volume of a storage or distribution medium, is called an "aggregate" if the copyright resulting from the compilation is not used to limit the legal rights of the compilation's users beyond what the individual works permit. When the Document is included in an aggregate, this License does not apply to the other works in the aggregate which are not themselves derivative works of the Document.

If the Cover Text requirement of section 3 is applicable to these copies of the Document, then if the Document is less than one half of the entire aggregate, the Document's Cover Texts may be placed on covers that bracket the Document within the aggregate, or the electronic equivalent of covers if the Document is in electronic form. Otherwise they must appear on printed covers that bracket the whole aggregate.

8. TRANSLATION

Translation is considered a kind of modification, so you may distribute translations of the Document under the terms of section 4. Replacing Invariant Sections with translations requires special permission from their copyright holders, but you may include translations of some or all Invariant Sections in addition to the original versions of these Invariant Sections. You may include a translation of this License, and all the license notices in the Document, and any Warranty Disclaimers, provided that you also include the original English version of this License and the original versions of those notices and disclaimers. In case of a disagreement between the translation and the original version of this License or a notice or disclaimer, the original version will prevail.

If a section in the Document is entitled "Acknowledgements", "Dedications", or "History", the requirement (section 4) to Preserve its Title (section 1) will typically require changing the actual title.

9. TERMINATION

You may not copy, modify, sublicense, or distribute the Document except as expressly provided for under this License. Any other attempt to copy, modify, sublicense or distribute the Document is void, and will automatically terminate your rights under this License. However, parties who have received copies, or rights, from you under this License will not have their licenses terminated so long as such parties remain in full compliance.

10. FUTURE REVISIONS OF THIS LICENSE

The Free Software Foundation may publish new, revised versions of the GNU Free Documentation License from time to time. Such new versions will be similar in spirit to the present version, but may differ in detail to address new problems or concerns. See http://www.gnu.org/copyleft/.

Each version of the License is given a distinguishing version number. If the Document specifies that a particular numbered version of this License "or any later version" applies to it, you have the option of following the terms and conditions either of that specified version or of any later version that has been published (not as a draft) by the Free Software Foundation. If the Document does not specify a version number of this License, you may choose any version ever published (not as a draft) by the Free Software Foundation.

INDEX

www.ingramcontent.com/pod-product-compliance
Lightning Source LLC
Chambersburg PA
CBHW072139270326
41931CB00010B/1812